EAT WELL, LOVE WELL

Eat Well, Love Well

By
Michael L. McCann, B.S., M. Div., Ed. D., N.D.

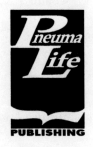

Eat Well, Love Well

By

Michael L. McCann, B.S., M. Div., Ed.D., N.D.

Unless otherwise noted, Scripture quotations are from the King James Version of the Bible. Scripture quotations marked NIV are taken from the New International Version of the Bible. Copyright V 1973, 1978, 1984 International Bible Society. Used by permission of Zondervan Bible Publishers.

Copyright © 2002 Michael L. McCann, B.S., M. Div., Ed.D., N.D.
ISBN 1-56229-163-7

Pneuma Life Publishing, Inc.
P.O. Box 885
Lanham, MD 20703
301-218-8928
www.pneumalife.com

Printed in the United States of America 1 3 5 7 9 10 8 6 4 2

Disclaimer

Much of the advice in this book is based upon the research, professional and personal experiences of the author. If the reader has any questions concerning any material or procedure mentioned, the author strongly suggests seeking the advise of a physician or professional health care practitioner. The advice of a health care practitioner as well as proper medical screening should precede the start of any new diet, supplement or treatment program. Some of the treatments and suggestions mentioned in this book may have different effects on different people. The author is not liable for any advise, effects or consequences resulting from the use or misuse of any procedures, materials or preparations suggested in this book. The author believes that this information can be helpful to the general public.

Contents

Introduction

Your Personal Domain

God has given us a unique situation, marriage, where covenant leads to a lifetime of commitment. All of us need to view our marriages in a very special way. Marriage is our personal domain where as loving couples we may experience the utmost in pleasure.

The purpose in writing this book is to lead Christian couples to find sexual fulfillment in their married state. It is totally based on Biblical principles that will bring greater results in lovemaking. The vitamins, minerals and herbs can only aid the married couple in finding greater fulfillment.

Your personal domain is your own little kingdom. Your own kingdom has a King and His name is the Lord Jesus Christ. Both you and your marriage partner must share the same commitment to the Lord if you are to experience total sexual bliss in the bedroom.

Your personal domain within marriage is that place where you are intimate with your mate in private, totally removed from public view, where the both of you experience and enjoy each other's bodies. This wonderful domain must be apart from the rush of everyday life. It must become a place of renewal and refreshment in each other's arms where you become one flesh just as God's Word promises. It is in this domain that you cautiously maintain the principles of privacy and experience oneness in the physical, emotional and spiritual realms.

Never take for granted the privacy of your personal domain. No matter how many vitamins or minerals you might be taking for better performance, life will bring its attacks against your marriage. Invasions such as financial pressures, illnesses and work-related stress do come from the outside world. If you have not totally surrendered to Jesus Christ, the attacks can destroy God's very best for you.

The worst attacks upon your marriage are the heart attitudes: pride, self-pity, anger, bitterness and resentment. Watch out for these because they can come from your best friends or even family members. Take great diligence in protecting your marriage and its domain.

The mind can only initiate what is being fed to it. If the mind is filled with Godly and good thoughts, then the greater the enjoyment will be that the body experiences. It is essential that the body as well as the mind be in good shape. The mind and body will work together if the chemical elements are in all the correct places at the right time. Thus, the nervous system, digestive system, circulatory system, glandular system, skeletal system, elimination system and muscular systems need proper nutrients to function for peak performance.

God has given us sex to experience it within marriage and to procreate the human race. The degree to which you enjoy sex will be primarily dependent upon your mind and thought life. It is so essential to have good, kind and tender thoughts in relationship to lovemaking. Consequently the more positive we can be in our thought life, especially concerning our mates, the better will be the enjoyment of intercourse.

It is impossible to experience true and lasting satisfaction if your life is filled with sin and out of order. That is, if you're not given to Jesus Christ. Great sex comes in marriage where the conditions are perfect in your private and personal domain. For all of this to happen, the spirit, soul and body need to be in harmony.

Taking care of your body by good nutrition, exercise, rest and vitamin supplementation will help you enter your private domain ready to experience God's best for each other. Sex can increase personal alertness and increase your mental faculties if the body has been taken care of properly.

Great sex in marriage will keep you young and joyful. Cherish and protect your personal domain since the quality of your relationship will bring greater commitment to each other and to Jesus Christ.

Your whole life can far exceed your wildest expectations if you follow the principles set down in this book. This humble book is only a guidebook. It will greatly enhance not only your love life but also life itself. I wish you the greatest possible joy in your lovemaking.

— *Michael L. McCann*

Chapter 1

To Attract or
Not To Attract!

There are universal laws that control the manner in which men and women are attracted to each other. This certainly may not seem very romantic, but I assure you that God has put it all together.

The Bible is full of information about sex and attraction. Almost every Book of the Bible speaks openly about joyous sex in marriage. The Song of Solomon exquisitely depicts a sexual relationship in marriage. In the Book of Genesis God shows us most implicitly what He has thought about marriage and love.

God has placed much emphasis on sexual union in marriage. The first three chapters of Genesis record how God created man and woman. It is clearly stated that "God saw everything that he had made, and, behold, it was very good" (Gen. 1:31). God created the light, and it was "good." The creations of land and sea were "good," and the creation of vegetation, of fish, and birds and animals were also "good." However, please note that it was not until the creation of man and woman that it was "very good."[1]

We know from psychology that there are two hemispheres of the brain: the left and right hemisphere. In part this maybe the reason that we are attracted to certain individuals rather than others. The left hemisphere of the brain functions as the rational, thinking and analytic side of the brain. The right hemisphere is involved with emotions, beauty, music and feelings. It is believed that men are more dominated by left-brain activity—problem solving or working with tools. On the other hand, it is believed that women are dominated by right-brain activity. Thus, women tend to socialize more than men do because they have greater artistic talents.

At the same time, both sexes have much in common such as strength, intelligence, love, hope and ambition. God has created us to complement each other, and yet each sex has qualities which are unique to that particular sex. For instance, most men tend to have trouble expressing sensitivity and feelings whereas most women tend to be sensitive and compassionate.

Beyond our physical attraction, it is necessary to work at bonding together. Relationships are progressive; that is, as we grow together we find we have things in common.

If a relationship is to last a lifetime, then we need to have common interests and likes. There must be mutual affinities that will enable the couple to grow and find each other's presence enjoyable. Without this, the infatuation stage of love will not be strong enough to sustain the relationship.

For the best success in a relationship, the couple needs to list their mutual likes and dislikes consciously. For instance, do they share similar goals and aspirations? Do they share similar hopes and attitudes? If a majority of their individual interests is not mutually agreed upon, then love will be difficult to sustain in the marriage. For example, say the wife likes classical music but the husband likes hard rock. They need to come to terms about these differences before marriage.

All of us need mates who will motivate and encourage us to grow and develop, not only in our personal talents, but also in things of the Lord. Marriage can be most enjoyable if both partners will work at having a good time and appreciate one another.

Christian marriage is a covenant in which couples will find completion in their mutual companionship. This companionship finds completion on the spiritual, mental and the physical levels during sexual intercourse. Understand that fulfillment in marriage is a two-way street. As we fulfill the needs of our marital partner, we too find fulfillment and completion in ourselves. It is good to know that love works through both the rational, analytical left-side brain and at the same time the right brain functions to find elements in another person that will bring fulfillment to the other person.[2]

Repressed love will lead to a shallow, meaningless existence. There is so much emphasis on sex today in our culture that our society has forgotten that sex focused in the wrong direction is destructive.

While emotions play a part in the initial attraction, emotions in and of themselves can never sustain a marriage. There are times in marriage when there will be bleak days, and during those times emotions may be most negative concerning our mate. If the marriage is based on faulty emotions there will be great strain, which could lead to divorce. Marriage must be based upon a bond of commitment that aids the husband or wife through the good times and the bad. Commitment is the needed ingredient that assists the couple in developing a greater love.

The way the person looks, smells and the sound of the voice can all be elements that will attract us to one another. Even the touch of the hand can be an element of attraction. All of these little things help us consciously or unconsciously in selecting a marital partner.

The things that initially attract us to one another can also change over the years as we get older and our appearance begins to change. Attraction in a marriage must be based upon mutual understanding of each other not just the physical. As partners work together, serve together and play together, they will be most happy. Working at having a good marriage makes happy marriages.

The practical function of sexual attractiveness is to bring a member of the opposite sex into your life for the possibility of marriage. God desires you to be physically attracted to one another. However, relationships based upon just sex will very seldom, if ever, become more than shallow marriages. Sex outside of marriage is sin, but even more dangerous are the numerous sexually transmitted diseases of today. The only safe sex that exists is within the confines of marriage.

Physical attractiveness must not be at the top of your priority list in selecting a mate. Take into consideration the whole person and not only what you see superficially as your criteria for selection of a future partner. Above all, pray about any possible future mate. Marriage partners need the counsel of the Holy Spirit before they stand before God.

Learning to hear the Holy Spirit about a possible marital partner is most important. Not knowing what God is saying about a mate will only bring heartache. Divorce happens to Christians because of not hearing what the Holy Spirit has to say about a future mate or because they're not waiting on God's timeline.

Make marriage count. As Christians, we need to show the world the goodness of God's covenant by living our lives to the fullest with dignity and sanctity. The dignity of marriage has been lost because of the world's interpretation of it. American culture has lost the meaning and dignity of God's great covenant called marriage by cheapening the marriage vows. When vows are exchanged before God and man, these vows are to last for a lifetime.

A Christ-centered marriage is aesthetic and totally wonderful. It is in understanding the Christian marriage relationship where God means for us to achieve total sexual satisfaction.

Chapter 2

Understanding Marriage

Marriage should be a joyous celebration of two people who join their hearts together in Christian love. As they live together as lovers, they experience great blessings in Christ and learn to grow together. Their relationship founded in Christ produces a fount of wisdom. When they experience Jesus in their marriage nothing can ever break them apart for they have become one in spirit, soul and body. Their personal intimacies extrude great joy, happiness and lasting friendship. They truly want to be together for the rest of their lives since they have found the secret of lasting happiness in Christ. Together they develop their gifts, talents and abilities. Each partner helps the other to become all he or she is meant to be in Christ.

Love in marriage is essential. It is totally giving to the other and not asking anything in return. Love does not contain the marriage but the marriage contains the love. Marital love should always be growing—not dying. As a couple lives together over the years, their experience of love may at times need rekindling. This can be done through weekends alone without the children and taking time out to get to know one another again.

There can be no better definition of love than 1 Corinthians 13:4-7: "Charity (love) suffereth long, and is kind, charity envieth not; charity vaunteth not itself, is not puffed up. Doth not behave itself unseemly, seeketh not her own, is not easily provoked, thinketh no evil; Rejoiceth not in iniquity, but rejoiceth in the truth; Beareth all things, believeth all things, hopeth all things, endureth all things."

Paul here is giving us a "behavioral definition" of love. He clearly describes how love behaves in personal relationships. This not only enables us to understand the nature of love, but also gives a clear criteria by which true spirituality may be evaluated.

The Bible speaks to us of another kind of love that only Christians can experience. This is found in the New Testament and it is called "agape" love. It is love experienced both in word and action. Agape love is unconditional and has a profound depth to it. This kind of love allows us to enjoy a true "one flesh" experience in marriage.

When Paul speaks of agape love, he is speaking about the love that is unconditional and irrevocable. This is the love that God gave to Christ our Lord-a love that lead Him to the cross for our sakes. This love is not found in the world because it is truly supernatural. It is love given out of joy seeking only the highest good for His creation. This wonderful love does not depend upon our actions toward God. He loves whether or not there is any response to it. God loves us unconditionally.

When there is true agape love in marriage, it can overcome all problems or circumstances. This glorious bond between a husband and wife can show them moments of enjoyment beyond anything previously anticipated.

The New Testament clearly teaches that agape love must be in the marriage which means a total commitment to each other. As God showed His total commitment to mankind by sending His son Jesus Christ into the world to save us from our sins, so we must be willing to give all to our partners in marriage.

Often times Christians allow worldly concepts to enter their marriage. The end product of all of this is a confused or mixed idea of love. The world has no clear understanding of the meaning of love because God *is* love and they don't know Him. For the world's view, love can be passion, affection, romantic feelings, friendships, fondness, infatuation. When the world speaks of love, it always means getting something in return. When the Bible speaks of love it always speaks of giving. "For God so loved the world that he gave His only begotten Son" (John 3:16).

The world must not dictate marital expectations to Christian couples. As God commanded Adam to "cleave" to Eve, so this same commitment must be made by both partners in marriage. As a man loves his mate, he must love her with all of his heart even before the marriage. This total commitment must be done on the part of both partners in order for the marriage to be successful.

With today's marriages of convenience, the idea of total commitment would appear to be out of date. Although the world accepts divorce as a normal everyday thing, there are people who still expect their marriages to last forever. The divorce rate in the United States is now in excess of 50 percent. This can only tell us that there is great misunderstanding of the meaning of commitment.

Jesus said, "What, therefore, God hath joined together, let no man put asunder" (Mark 10:9). This verse needs to be impressed deeply upon our minds. This means a total commitment to the marriage no matter what may transpire. Couples today must enter marriage with the preconceived notion that there is no way out for them. With this in mind, both partners will be committed in making a success of the marriage.

Many couples come to the point where they admit, "We have lost our love for each other" but what they are actually saying is that the marriage is over. This only confirms that they never had the agape love in the first place. They have confused "feeling" with true love. When love is based upon feelings, the end result in marriage is divorce. When a marriage is built on feelings, every time there is a change of circumstances, the marriage becomes more shaky.

Emotions will never sustain a marriage. As the commitment binds a husband and wife together through the various trials, tribulations and joys, their agape love will increase. Commitment is a bond of which good feelings emerge because there is a Christian commitment in every situation.

Hollywood portrays a glamorous woman swept away by a tall, handsome, young man who live happily ever after. Their world is free of hard work, worry and even anxiety. There is always a flurry of kisses and sexual intimacy. Most of us should realize that this is fantasy and not the real world. Real love costs a couple a great deal of time and energy. Marriage is an institution that requires diligence and hard work in every area-including sex.

Most of our concepts of life and love are formulated during our teen years. As this is so, it is not difficult to see that even Christians divorce since their concepts of Christian marriage have not been thoroughly thought out. Especially if our attitudes toward life and love are not Christ-centered, personal relationships will disintegrate later on in life.

When teenagers have been taught that the body and sexual feelings are somehow unclean or worthless, these negative attitudes will show up in later life. These beliefs may help encourage a higher spirituality, but they cause untold mental anguish down the road. God does not disapprove our bodies since He made them in His image.

Part of the reason we need to work hard at our sex life is not because of technique or pleasure, but rather to improve our self-image.

Unfortunately, the biggest misrepresentation of our self-image comes from worldly advertisements. From an early age, we are bombarded through the media with a perfect image. The truth is, while a certain level of healthfulness is good, it's impossible to attain the world's concept of perfection.

This is the only body you're going to get this side of heaven. God wants you to love your body just as it is regardless of whether it is perfect or not. He made our bodies in His image, and since He doesn't disapprove, why should we? The human body is the house of the spirit, and the spirit comes with the body. You will never be happy trying to be someone else. Be comfortable with the body that God has given you.

You really can't love someone else until you've first learned to love yourself. If an individual is occupied with how they look all of the time, it becomes most difficult to accept the love of someone else. This encourages the belief that they are just not "loveable." When the individual is told how beautiful she actually is, this creates a problem of trust in her life. This negative emotion gets in the way of our ability to love or receive love from the person who has complimented us.

When you're in love with another, you begin to share the same language and understanding, and you experience true oneness. Mature, true love sees the needs of the other above its own needs. When that spark is ignited, the couple begins to not to see the short comings or faults of the other, rather they focus on the positive attributes.

Mature love is more than just a physical or biological function. Mature love is just as powerful a force as sex but in a different manner. Unlike sex, mature love does not have the sense of urgency about it as sex does.

God created sex for pleasure which is to be contained in marriage. We are fashioned to take pleasure in our bodies and these feelings that are associated with our sexuality. Both love and pleasure will find total freedom and bliss as partners share their bodies in the marriage bed.

Sex itself is most pleasurable but sex has maximized potential and is more desirable within the marriage covenant. God has so ordained the covenant of marriage so that the couple might experience true sexual bliss.

Unfortunately with the pace of life as it is today, many couples have never achieved their maximum sexual potential. God has not designed us to experience sexual bliss in a hurry. Godly wisdom is needed to have a healthy sex life. In order to have a healthy sex life, we need to be healthy-spirit, soul (mind) and body.

We neglect our health and abuse our bodies with drugs, alcohol and refined foods. If we really cared about our bodies, we would not saturate the air with nicotine or tars from cigarettes and exercise would be pursued with a greater enthusiasm. The realization that most diseases can be prevented by participating in exercise activities would encourage us to do more.

American Christians are killing themselves by making poor choices of foods. Our very culture encourages us to make these choices in the selections of foods, drinks and lack of exercise. It's most difficult to have good sex when you're forty or fifty pounds overweight. Our country is a nation of overweight people who refuse to take the time to understand what it is they are doing to their bodies.

Once we learn to maximize our health and not neglect our bodies, then we will learn the secret to a great sex life.

We can change our faulty diets into healthy eating patterns that last a lifetime.

Chapter 3

Our Faulty Diets

Diet is so very important in having a good emotional and sex life. Yes, it is correct; what you eat will either foster good health or tear it down. It is difficult to have good sex when you're constantly tired or feeling poorly, because the body chemistry is out of balance and needs to be brought into proper balance so that the joy of living will return once again.

Never have we ever lived in such a day as this one! Our food is literally filled with chemical additives. People are dying needlessly because our livers are loaded with all kinds of chemicals that have been put into our foods. These chemicals will affect our moods and even our personalities. Consequently, they will definitely affect our sex lives.

Our water, air and soil have been filled with pollutants over the years which have aided in the breakdown of the health of this nation. Coffee, tea, alcohol and nicotine are the most widely used drugs in America today. Each of these has a negative influence on anyone's sex life.

At the same time, there are those chemical imbalances that are brought about by stress and poor diet. This does not take into consideration the problems countless Americans experience from constipation.

As Christians, we need to come to the point where we must make better choices of just how to live a good healthy life. Our lives will never be normal until we give up the use of drugs and the countless wrong food choices that are made every day at the grocery store. There is a way out of our love and sex problems, but it is going to take time to get your body right again. Remember it took years to create the problem and it will take a considerable amount of effort and time to change your lifestyle.

We live in a most stressful society, which in turn affects our emotions. For example, when anger is at work in the body, it sets off a chemical chain reaction in the body. Through many years of practice I have seen that people who are always angry and full of condemnation have made very wrong choices in relationship to the food they eat. Negative emotions foster poor health. People who are constantly negative have unhealthy diets and unhealthy ways of living. There is a better way of living if we will choose it. Living a natural lifestyle will definitely improve your over all health.

Good Mind, Good Lovin'

Good love begins in the mind. It is estimated that 90 percent of sex is in the mind. If this is the case, can you see the need for balancing the emotional life with good godly thoughts and aspirations? When this is done there will be a definite improvement in your ability to function in the bedroom. Good lovemaking must be done in a mood of peacefulness. If there is stress or a rush about doing things, the end result will not be as nearly as good. As you think, so you become.

The hypothalamus is a portion of the diencephalon of the brain. This portion of the brain activates, controls and stimulates the peripheral autonomic nervous system, endocrine processes and many somatic functions, such as body temperature, sleep and appetite.[1] The hypothalmus has the ability of receiving nerve messages from that part of the brain that functions as the thinking part. It also acts as a central switchboard for the emotional centers of the brain and from all the organs, glands and tissues of the human body. It also triggers nerve impulses helping in balancing the body's own chemistry. The hypothalamus functions in the body assisting the endocrine glands. The sex center is found here in this marvelous portion of the brain.

Therefore, if the mind is not at peace the body chemistry will not be at peace. It is impossible to live in anger, bitterness, hatred and resentment without reaping both the physical and spiritual consequences of such powerful destructive emotions. Naturally the sex life is going to pay a price with detrimental effects. The body chemistry will be totally affected causing needless suffering and even disease.

The apostle Paul tells us in Ephesians 5:28, "Husbands, love your wives, even as Christ also loved the church, and gave himself for it." We need to love, care for and cherish our mates. We must have the proper attitude toward them and not allow ourselves to be overtly critical toward them. If we are to have great sex with them, it is necessary to assist them in personal growth and advancement. Above all, we need to allow our partners the right of becoming all that God wants them to be.

As I tell young couples in premarital counseling, "Don't try to change your mate, it's a total waste of time. But do try to change yourself." Each of us must be an example to the other and then change will take place. As this new understanding becomes a part of your daily thinking your love life will improve. The chemicals within your body will become more harmonized both on the physical as well psychological aspect of lovemaking.[2]

In 1925 Dr. Hans Selye, a European physician trained at the German University at Prague, noticed that most of his patients had certain common symptoms. Those symptoms were: fatigue, aching bones and joints, loss of appetite and even weight. From this he was able to conclude a concept of stress that could be found worldwide. His theory of stress included the body's ability of "wear-and-tear caused by just living." He explains the role of such agents as intoxication, trauma, nervous strain, heat, cold, muscular fatigue, polluted air and radiation.[3]

Dr. Selye explains that the body reacts to stress in the same way it reacts to danger by going through a series of biochemical changes. We know it as "fight or flight," but he entitled it the General Adaptation Syndrome (GAS).[4] He calls the first stage the "alarm reaction." The body begins to mobilize its natural defenses against the cause of the stress (stressor agent). Nerve impulses from the brain are sent to the adrenal medulla to secrete adrenalin and other stress related hormones. Cortisol is one that, if found too often in the body, can actually cause the burn-out of the adrenal glands. Thus, the "fight or flight" response. The heart beat is accelerated, blood pressure levels become elevated, and an increased amount of blood flows to the muscles and the lungs dilate to increase the respiratory effort.

Dr. Selye called the second stage of the General Adaption Syndrome the "resistance" phase. This is the phase where the body continues to fight the stressor long after the effects of the "fight or flight" response have worn off.[5] If the stress is caused by infective agents, the body's immune system will increase its activity. If the stress should be physical, the neuroendocrine system converts the body's own protein to ready energy. If the stress is psychological, there will occur a combination of responses, such as anxiety and shortness of breath.[6]

The third stage of the General Adaptation Syndrome is "exhaustion." This is the result of the prolongation of the resistance reaction or continue stress leading to total "burnout."

The exhaustion may manifest itself in a total malfunction of various body organs or even all body systems. Continued stress overworks the heart, blood vessels, adrenals and the immune system. If the stress is overwhelming, general depression will ensue. Also, low blood pressure, increased heart rate, increased cortisol (natural steroid hormone), and low sex steroid hormone secretions occur as a result of stress.[7]

Now that we have examined some of the physiological factors involved in stress, can we not see why lovemaking and good sex often times are boring rather than interesting? This is why the utmost care must be taken to protect us from every-day stress that is disastrous toward a good sex life.

At the same time we have discovered many things about the way foods, drugs and alcohol alter our moods. Nutritionists now know that a niacin deficiency can encourage depression as well as food allergies and low blood sugar.

Endorphins, a brain chemical, have been found to reduce pain in the body and create an overall feeling of wellness. Endorphins are able to create a natural "high," which is certainly better than using drugs to achieve the same result. Various endocrine glands release hormones that may produce feelings of well being, sexual arousal and alertness. These same hormones have the ability to influence metabolism positively or negatively.

Since our hormones definitely affect our feelings of "falling in love," we need to know that what we eat, drink or even smell can greatly influence our love lives. These factors can alter our body chemistry, which will directly affect our soulish emotions.

God has designed us so that we are not truly satisfied with simply physical and psychological release in sex. With God's perfect design, a marriage filled with agape love will encourage greater emotions of love and intimacy. Emotions and feelings play a profound part of good sex, but agape love in a marriage the framework of commitment. Our emotions can change hour by hour as we allow our hormones to influence us. There will be times when physical desire for your partner may be paramount, and that's fine. However, there are other times when only affection and close companionship are desired for that moment. Sexual desire may arise only after much time spent together releasing pent-up stress from the day's labor. If we have centered our lives in Christ, we will experience a blessed assurance with our partners in the midst of perplexing changes all around us. Remember, the best sex you will ever experience in marriage will be God's kind of love.

Changing Your Lifestyle

Many emotional problems that occur in marriage may be related to the problem of unhealthy blood. Consider this for a moment. When an individual eats all processed foods, drinks alcohol, coffee and tea, which are all lifeless foods, how can good health be encouraged? When food is lifeless, demineralized, devitaminized, refined and bleached, it is certain that it will not foster good health. It becomes most obvious that if couples want good sex they have to eat God's way.

Christians want miracles of healing. I know this because my wife, Rita, and I have been involved in a healing ministry for over twenty years. People want instant miracles and healings. At the same time, they are not truly willing to change their lifestyles. How can they erase all their ills when they keep breaking important and vital health laws? We should understand that what we eat and drink today will affect our walk and talk tomorrow. If we fill ourselves with "junk food," is it any wonder that after some years of marriage that sex becomes rather difficult at times? Only a clear thinking person will make sure what he puts in his stomach will contribute to health and long life.

When disease strikes the human body, many people cry out in pain and anguish, but their condition is the result of poor eating habits. There are numerous factors in their lives that affect them negatively, thus the end result is poor sex in marriage because the joy is gone.

To become a healthy lover, we have to make a lifestyle change. When we eliminate all those negative things, then we are able to become more healthy and better lovers.

Ask yourself the following questions:

1. Do you spend time with your mate in prayer? Are you attending church together? Who is the head of your house?

2. Check out the food that you are eating. How many fresh foods do you consume each day? Do you eat raw vegetables each day?

3. Attempt to practice walking in divine health. Eat as naturally as you are able. Avoid medication as much as possible.

4. Check out all of your relationships. If they are destructive or critical, seek our Lord in prayer so that they may be healed or ended.

5. Find gainful employment that you will really like. Make sure that the atmosphere is conducive to foster good relationships.

6. Spend family time with your children. Pray with your children.

7. Be in a church where you feel comfortable. Try to have an active part in the life of the church.

8. Commit yourself totally to Jesus Christ. Practice loving people and make it your goal to be kind and generous to all!

9. Know your strong points and weak points. Never allow yourself to be taken advantage of even if the other person is a Christian.

10. Do not tolerate in your mind negative thoughts. Never even think of getting divorced. This word should not be in your vocabulary.

This questionnaire is simply to help you consider where you are in life and where you want to go. Whether your lifestyle changes or not is up to you.

Chapter 4

Minerals Make Things Work Better

Part of correcting a faulty diet and alternating our lifestyle is receiving the proper minerals in the correct amounts. Unfortunately, we do not hear enough about minerals and their importance in our diet. Most other types of nutrients have stolen the spotlight in the pursuit of glorious health and personality improvement. God has given us minerals to make the difference in good health and even in good sex. Without minerals, all other nutrients would be useless.

Minerals are needed for overall mental and physical functioning. Minerals are essential in maintaining proper physiological conditions and processes, such as the acid-base balance, osmotic action, elasticity and soft tissues such as muscles.[1] The integrity of the skeletal structure's strength depends upon these magic minerals. Nerves need minerals to be tranquil, strong and vibrant. Even the function of digestion needs sufficient "mineralization" to function in the assimilation and breakdown of foods. Minerals are found in all tissues and fluids, but more especially in bones, teeth and cartilage.[2]

There are close to thirty minerals that help in the maintenance of health and even prevent premature aging by helping to preserve youthful vigor in the nerves, muscles, heart, hair, blood, brain and other bodily attributes.

D. T. Quigley, M.D., in *Magic Minerals,* declares:

We do know that the person who has a sufficient intake of calcium, iron and iodine...(plus vitamins) will have a resistance against ordinary disease in excess of the average person. Such persons will have more freedom from fatigue and greater ability to work; will live with retention of all physical faculties to a greater age, and will have a better mind than the person who suffers from some single or multiple vitamin or mineral deficiency. The various vitamins and minerals are all necessary. No one can be omitted if an individual would retain good health."[3]

Minerals, when taken in proper dosages, have the unique power of maintaining a delicate internal water balance that is needed for all mental and physical processes. Minerals aid in keeping blood and tissue fluids from becoming either too acid or too alkaline.[4] Minerals stimulate the hormonal secretion of glands and cause the nervous system to mentally communicate to various parts of the human body.

The body needs minerals to serve as detoxifying (purifying) agents by joining with acid wastes from the cells of the body. Minerals neutralize these wastes and get them ready for elimination. If this did not take place, waste products would decompose and make you sluggish, sleepy, ache, nervous, grouchy and an unpleasant person to be around.

Minerals work to equalize the amount of dissolved solids both within and outside the cells. Consequently, internal and external pressures are equalized and the body's cells remain in perfect homeostasis. This process is known as "osmotic equilibrium," a condition of superb youthful health that requires a balance of sufficient mineral supply.

Your blood and lymph are liquids in which solids are kept in solution.[5] Cells are always being washed in lymph fluids. Our cells are semi-fluid containing dissolved matter.

If the lymph outside your cells contain as much dissolved solid as found within the cells, you run the risk of having your body's cells shrink and even dissolve! If you have more dissolved solid inside your cells than dissolved solid outside, it is possible that your cells could bloat up and even burst! When this condition is existent, this condition turns a calm person into a nervous one. This condition leads to short tempers, irritation, tension and premature aging. A happy, healthy and even-tempered person is one who has a balance of his internal fluids. His minerals are in proper proportion.

A person who is mineral-rich is a happy, successful person, radiating a personality so vibrant, different and unusual that you instinctively admire him. Minerals will influence an individual's behavior. Minerals strengthen your nerves, give you a sharp mind, banish jitters and put a glow in your skin and a sparkle in your eyes.

Minerals act as catalysts that make possible the function of enzymes; they form the structure upon which the body is built. When minerals are sufficient they make possible a healthy, strong body. When there is a deficiency of minerals, their absence may result in disturbances of a most serious nature. They can make or break your body. Consequently, we can see how they are needed in proper proportion for a good sex life.

Mineral deficiency can lead to a retarded birth rate, goiter, anemia and poor digestion. Your climate may be perfect—the weather warm and the sun shiny—but if your diet is low in the minerals your body needs, you could still suffer disease.

Minerals, in adequate amounts, will help keep the body young. There are close to thirty such minerals that help prevent premature aging by helping to preserve youthful stamina in the nerves, muscles, heart, blood, glands and the brain. Minerals also help support the immune system. In addition, adequate amounts of minerals will help reduce fatigue and give greater strength for work. When individuals have sufficient minerals in their diets, they can mature with all physical faculties to greater age and will have a sharper mind than the person who suffers from single or multiple vitamin or minerals deficiency.[6]

Minerals have numerous important functions within the body. The main functions they perform are as follows:

1. The building blocks of our bodies, which is protein, are formed only in the presence of calcium, nitrogen and sulphur.

2. The entire digestive system is dependent upon potassium to cause proper function of the vagus nerve, which is a nerve found in the stomach and aids in digestion.

3. Many vitamins are totally dependent upon minerals for their functioning.

4. Minerals are necessary with vitamins to remove internal gaseous waste products. It is a fact that individuals suffering from multiple sclerosis suffer from damage to the nerve covering caused by an excess of a carbon-nitrogen substance. It is thought that prevention of this diseased condition or removal of the harmful substance can be accomplished if the body is properly fed with minerals, especially cobalt.[7]

5. Since the insulin molecule contains zinc, and since diabetes results from an insulin shortage, it is thought that a deficiency of zinc mineral is involved with this disease.

6. Minerals influence muscle contraction and are essential for nerve response.

7. Minerals function to control body liquids and permit other nutrients to pass into the bloodstream. Without minerals, other nutrients are not able to do their job as they should.

8. Blood coagulation is dependent upon mineral action. Bruises, cuts, scratches and wounds need minerals for the healing process.

9. Personal alertness, youthful energy and thought power all require minerals such as manganese, copper, cobalt, iodine, zinc, magnesium and phosphorous for utmost efficiency.

10. Minerals in our bloodstream assist in creating a germ-killing action. Minerals have an antibiotic function within the bloodstream provided other essential raw materials are also present.

11. Minerals are necessary for strong bones and teeth, which are composed of about 95 percent calcium and phosphorous.[8]

Glorious health can come to us if we are eating healthy fresh food and taking needed supplements.

Fourteen Incredible Minerals and How They Can Help You

The need of calcium in the American diet cannot be stressed enough. We are a people who are becoming calcium depleted. For calcium to be effective and to function properly, we must have vitamins D, A, C and phosphorus. These other vitamins must also have calcium for them to do the work that what is intended for them. About 99 percent of calcium is found in bones and teeth, the other estimated 1 percent circulates in your body fluids and tissues. Calcium is necessary for blood clotting, to activate enzymes (digestive juices), and to control and regulate the passage of fluids throughout the cellular walls.

Calcium works to normalize the contraction and the relaxation of your heart. If a person's blood level of calcium should drop, he becomes nervous and irritated. An adequate calcium intake means that some is kept on reserve in the ends of the bones in long, needle-like crystals called *trabeculate*. This is needed so that when the body is in stress, this maybe called upon and used. If calcium is insufficient, then the body takes calcium out of the bone structure, usually the spinal and pelvic bones.

Calcium is necessary for the protection of the acid/alkaline balance, which affects the production of hormones by the endocrine glands. Calcium helps regulate the menstrual cycle and the fertility of both men and women.[9] Without calcium in abundance the nerves and muscles are greatly affected.

Calcium does indeed affect the sex life of all individuals. It has the propensity of steadiness of affection, protects from over-excitement and gives strength during the performance of sexual intercourse. Calcium helps to keep emotions under control. Calcium insufficiency can reduce the sexual interest and led to poor performance.[10]

Studies have shown that women need 1,000 mg. of calcium daily to prevent osteoporosis. Osteoporosis is a calcium-deficiency disease characterized by poor bone porosity.[11] This is more noticeable after menopause.

When white sugar is ingested, it causes acidity in the body. Sodium, potassium, and calcium neutralize this affect. If calcium and sodium are short in the diet, calcium is then deposited in the joints as spurs and bumps.[12]

Good sources of natural calcium are yogurt, cheese, milk, salmon, dark green leafy vegetables (especially collard or turnip), legumes, broccoli and tofu. Although a known source of calcium, the problem with milk is that it is pasteurized and homogenized. These two processes alter the calcium in the milk and become very difficult to digest.

Goat milk is perhaps the best since it is rich in calcium and easily digested.

Phosphorus

Phosphorus is found in all of your body cells. It is estimated that 66 percent of body phosphorus is in our bones in the form of calcium phosphate. The other 33 percent is in soft tissue as organic and inorganic phosphate. This wonderful mineral converts oxidative energy to cell work. Phosphorus is known to influence proteins, carbohydrate and fat synthesis. In addition, it stimulates muscular contraction, secretion of glandular hormones, nerve impulses and kidney functioning.[13]

Phosphorus:

- ignites internal energy in the body
- works to neutralize excess body acidity
- stimulates the production of lecithin and cerebrin, ingredients needed for mental power and agility
- assists in metabolizing fats and starches.

It is believed that many overweight people may not have sufficient phosphorus in their diets. A deficiency of this trace mineral could cause appetite and weight loss or gain, nervous disorders, mental sluggishness and general fatigue. In extreme cases, there is irregularity in breathing and the individual appears to be pale and have a wan appearance.[14]

It is estimated that as much as 80 percent of the male sex fluid is lecithin. Lecithin acts as part of the nerve coating in the brain that prevents toxins and enhances nerve transmission.

Good sources of phosphorus and lecithin for the brain, glands and nerves are egg yolks, codfish roe, seafood, and raw milk products. Meat is a good source of phosphorus if it is not over cooked. Fried eggs lose all phosphorus so boiled and poached eggs are best.

Other good sources of phosphorus are from seeds, nuts, whole grains, rice polishings, wheat bran, legumes, cabbage, corn and other vegetable sources are more than adequate.[15]

Iron

Billions of body cells need iron for life-giving oxygen. Without iron in our diets, we would need about three hundred quarts of blood in our bodies just to survive. Because of sufficient iron in our blood, all we need is about six quarts of blood to sustain us. Iron is needed to form hemoglobin, the oxygen carrier in our blood. Iron influences the synthesis of proteins. At the same time, iron must have calcium and other nutrients in order to function properly. Iron is necessary in the blood but it is also present in enzymes that take part in cell respiration.

Without proper levels of iron in the blood, the ensuing problem of anemia is created. Anemia causes unnecessary fatigue and loss of interest in sex. Iron-rich blood creates that "sexy feeling."[16] It is basic in the production of body energy.

Only a small portion of iron is absorbed into the bloodstream. There must be other trace minerals such as copper, manganese and cobalt in foods for proper use by the body. Vitamin C plays a role in iron absorption. Good sources of iron includes red meats, egg yolks, green leafy vegetables, almonds, asparagus, fish, poultry, black raspberries, bing cherries, prunes, raisins and apricots.[17]

Iodine

For many decades it has been known that when there is a deficiency of iodine a goiter will form on the thyroid gland.

Today we know that this mineral is necessary in building intelligence. We have about 25 milligrams of iodine in our system. Two-thirds (15 milligrams) is in the thyroid gland, and the other one-third may be found in other parts of the body.

Iodine stimulates the thyroid to secrete the thyroxin hormone that regulates metabolism and energy levels. An iodine deficiency is characterized by goiter, obesity, sluggish metabolism and even slow thinking.

Other characteristics of an iodine deficiency will cause impairment of the mind and body, slow mental reaction and dry hair that easily breaks. Other symptoms will include rapid pulse, heart palpitation, tremors, nervousness, restlessness and increased irritability.

Iodine is essential for fat metabolism and other nutrients to function correctly. Iodine is abundant in all seafood and vegetables grown in iodine-rich soils. A most excellent source of iodine is kelp. Kelp is dehydrated seaweed. Kelp is available in most health stores, pharmacies and some special food shops. Another good source of iron is onions. Onions should be eaten as often as possible because of their medicinal properties.

Sodium

Sodium works with potassium to help maintain the favorable acid-base factor in the human body. It is needed to maintain a normal water level balance between cells and fluids. Sodium enables the nerves to respond to stimulation and transmit it. In addition to this, sodium gives strength to the muscles so they can contract. Sodium joins with chlorine to improve blood and lymph health. Its main function is to render other blood minerals more soluble and prevent them from becoming clogged or deposited in the circulatory system.

Good sources of sodium are seafood, poultry, beets, carrots, chard and dandelion greens. Perhaps the best source of sodium that is readily available and good for you is celery.

Potassium

Potassium is another "balancing" mineral. Potassium works synergistically with sodium to help normalize the rhythm of the heart and feed the muscular system. It joins with phosphorus to assist in sending oxygen to the brain. Sodium and potassium must be in balance. Sodium is found basically in the fluids circulating outside your cells and only a very small amount is found inside the cells. Potassium is found inside the cells and a small supply appears outside of the cells.

Potassium is needed for kidney stimulation to dispose of body wastes. Blood also requires potassium. A deficiency may cause constipation, nervous disorders, insomnia, slow and irregular heartbeat and even muscle damage. When there isn't sufficient potassium, the kidneys will enlarge and bones become brittle. Potassium directly affects human sexuality by insuring good nerve and muscle activity. Potassium maintains the right acid/alkaline balance for the production of hormones in the endocrine glands.

Potassium may be found in bananas, watercress, mint leaves, green pepper and chicory. Blackstrap molasses and figs contain large amounts of potassium.[18]

Magnesium

Magnesium is closely related to both calcium and phosphorus in its location and functioning in the human body. Nearly 70 percent of magnesium is found in the bones of the body. The rest may be found in the soft tissues and blood. It should be noted that muscle tissue contains more magnesium than calcium. Magnesium acts as a chemical starter for many reactions in the body. There is evidence between magnesium and the hormone cortisone as they affect the amount of phosphate in the blood.[19]

People with low levels of magnesium react to sound by becoming very nervous and often give exaggerated responses to even small noises or disturbances. When magnesium is supplied in the correct amount, many of these symptoms will disappear within a very short time.

Since magnesium acts as a muscle relaxer it has a definite role in lovemaking. Since many of our lifestyles are very active today and full of stress, this magnificent mineral can help in reducing stress in our lives. Magnesium will help stressful people to find relaxation and relief from tension. Having healthy levels of magnesium helps us to relax and allows us to focus on pleasing our partners instead of being absorbed about our performance level in bed.

Natural sources of magnesium include nuts, beans, peas, whole-grain breads, cereal, soybeans and dark green, leafy vegetables.[20]

Manganese

Manganese is a mineral that works with the B-complex vitamins to help over fatigue, sterility and poor sexual performance. It also combines with phosphatase (an enzyme) to build strong bones and teeth. Manganese is abundant in beef liver. This mineral is necessary for good enzymatic function so foods can be digested and vital nutrients extracted for over all body usage. Manganese helps strengthen the immune system and strong nerve health. In the expectant mother, manganese promotes milk formation.[21]

Chlorine

Chlorine acts like a broomstick in the human body by cleaning out toxic waste products from the digestive system. The liver is stimulated by chlorine so various waste products are eliminated through the bowels. Chlorine stimulates production of hydrochloric acid for the digestion of fibrous materials. In addition to this, chlorine helps in keeping a youthful joint and tendon conditions. It aids in the distribution of endocrine hormones.

When chlorine is insufficient, it may cause hair and teeth loss, poor muscular contractibility and poor digestive function. Chlorine may be found in kelp, dulse, sea greens, leafy greens, rye flour and ripened olives.[22]

Fluorine

Fluorine does help strengthen teeth enamel, but this is a tricky mineral. Too much of this mineral may actually cause abnormal and unsightly looking teeth. Miniscule amounts are found through the human body. When this mineral is taken in excess, it will actually weaken teeth and bones. It can be devastating to the internal organs when it is in excess.[23]

Zinc

Not only is zinc a constituent of insulin, but it is also part of the male reproductive fluid that is so necessary for proper functioning of the prostate and producing male hormones. It is made in the pancreas (a large gland located behind the lower part of the stomach) where it assists in the storage of glycogen, an energy producing substance. If this mineral is not adequate in the diet it will cause fatigue and a lethargic reaction.

Zinc works synergistically with phosphorus to aid in respiration, and it is needed in releasing the energy contained in vitamins. Zinc assists in respiration, and is related to carbohydrate utilization. Insulin is dependent upon zinc for the breaking down of sugars. Zinc also helps in the absorption of food through the intestinal walls. Zinc is present in lean meats and green leafy vegetables.[24]

Sulphur

Sulphur is the trace mineral that nature uses to make us "beautiful." Sulphur helps keep the hair glossy and smooth, aids the skin in keeping the complexion smooth and youthful, and invigorates the bloodstream, rendering it more powerful to resist many strains of bacterial infection.

When sulphur is present in the body it causes the liver to secrete bile, maintain over all body balance and influences the power of the brain. Sulphur works in conjunction with the B-complex vitamins that are needed for metabolism and good nerve health.

Sulphur may be found in fish, eggs, cabbage, lean beef and dried beans.[25]

Silicon

When the trace mineral silicon is deficient there will be noticeable skin flabbiness, a feeling of chronic fatigue and eyes that are dull and often appear glazed. The hair, muscles, nails, cellular walls and connective tissues all contain trace amount of silicon.

Silicon gives us the ability to get up and get going in our everyday lives. The sheaths of our nerves throughout the body and brain cannot be in good repair without this element. Good sources of silicon may be found in buckwheat products, mushrooms, carrots, tomatoes and liver.[26] Algae is also a good source of silicon.

Trace Elements (Micronutrients)

Chromium is a trace mineral that aids in regulating blood sugar level that determines available energy.[27] We know that many people living in the northern states suffer from chromium deficiencies since the soil is deplete of this trace mineral. Some of the excellent sources of this most important trace mineral is seafood, meats, whole grains and corn oil.

Germanium is a trace mineral about which very little is known. We do know that germanium does alleviate mood disorders that are directly related to our sex drive. It also enhances the immune system and does improve the function of the bowels. Good sources of germanium are found in green leaf vegetables, garlic, ginseng, aloe vera and comfrey.

Selenium is a most important trace mineral needed in conjunction with vitamin E to help create fertility and delay the oxidation of unsaturated fatty acids.[28] Good sources of selenium are whole wheat grains, fish, carrots, cabbage and Brazil nuts.

God has given us these most wonderful minerals to make our lives full of good health. If you want to spice up your sex life, make sure you are not mineral deficient.

Chapter 5

God-given Vitamins for a Joyous Sex Life

All of us want to have a joyous sex life and this is pos sible if we cooperate with God and His natural plan for good health. It is possible to be sexually active our entire lifetime if we follow God's plan for good health and long life. Vitamins are a vital part of good health and can change our overall health for the better.

Information—and misinformation—abounds about vitamins. Natural vitamins are organic food substances that may be found in plants and animals. Twenty substances have been discovered that are considered active in human nutrition, and these God-given vitamins are found in various degrees within specific foods, which are absolutely essential for natural growth and maintenance of good health. By in large, the body is unable to synthesize vitamins so they need to be provided in the diet or by food supplements.

Vitamins must have enzymes, which are chemicals, to perform numerous necessary functions within the body. Chemical enzymes consist of two parts: a protein molecule and a coenzyme. The coenzyme usually is a vitamin, or it may only contain part of a vitamin. Also, it could be a molecule that has been manufactured from a vitamin. Oxidation begins as the oxygen enters the bloodstream and travels to the cells where oxidation than takes place. Enzymes function as catalysts, which start the reactions that allow other materials to continue their work.

Regeneration in the body and the body chemistry often takes months. Continued vitamin supplementation will correct any deficiencies within the body and aid in regeneration. Over indulgence in vitamins will cause toxicity.

Scientists do not exactly know how vitamins work in the human body. They do know that they make a great difference in the overall health of an individual. Consequently, this will affect our sex lives. Many so called sex problems can be directly related to vitamin deficiencies. When the necessary supplements have been provided, many of these problems disappear. It is best to get our vitamins from the foods we eat, but often times the foods we ingest are not sufficient in vitamin content. Therefore, we need to take some supplements. Now let's take the time to look into vitamins and what they do for us.

Vitamin A

Vitamin A is a fat-soluble vitamin and is stored in the liver. We obtain some vitamin A from animal fats and the body makes part of it in the human intestine from beta-carotene and other carotenoids in fruits and vegetables. This is also present in the body in various chemical forms called retinoids, which aid in vision. So carrots really are good for the eyes!

Vitamin A will prevent night blindness. It also maintains the integrity of the skin and cells that line the respiratory and gastrointestinal tracts. It helps build strong teeth and bones and is essential for good reproductive health and normal growth. Vitamin A is essential for the immune

system and for the cells that line the airways and digestive tract.

Sources of vitamin A are found in fish, fish liver oils, liver, animal fat, eggs, cheese and yogurt.[1] Good sources of vitamin A are often found in fruits and vegetables that are orange or yellow in color. There are various herbs such as dandelion, parsley, mint and alfalfa, which are good sources of this vitamin.

When there is a deficiency of this vitamin, infection and inflammation can occur. There must be a word of caution about this vitamin. You must not exceed 25,000 I.U. a day as this amount can cause serious liver disease. Both vitamin E and zinc help the absorption of this vitamin.

Vitamin B

The B-complex vitamins help to maintain good health of the nerves, skin, eyes, hair, liver and mouth as well as the healthy muscle tone in the gastrointestinal tract. B vitamins are necessary for the good functioning of the brain. B-complex vitamins are coenzymes that function to create energy and is useful in alleviating depression and anxiety. It is necessary to take the B vitamins together. Taking a certain B vitamin for a period of time can cause damage to various parts of the body. To maintain the integrity of the B vitamin needed, always take the B-complex with the specific B vitamin that you are using.

Vitamin B-1 is called *thiamine.* Thiamine enhances circulation and assists in blood formation and carbohydrate metabolism. It assists in the production of hydrochloric acid, which is necessary for proper digestion. A deficiency of this vitamin will cause a person to feel lifeless, resulting in a diminished sex life.

When vitamin B-1 is not present, a nervous system disease known as Beriberi is formed. Other symptoms that result from a thiamine deficiency may include constipa-

Eat Well, Love Well

tion, edema, enlarged liver, fatigue, forgetfulness, gastrointestinal disturbances, muscle atrophy and numbness of hands and feet.[2]

Good sources of thiamine are raw nuts and seeds, especially sunflower seeds. Asparagus, beans, pineapple, soy beans, yogurt, wheat germ, whole wheat, brown rice and other whole grains are food products that will give ample amounts of thiamine. Liver, lean meat and fish are animal sources of thiamine.

Vitamin B-2 is essential for red blood cell formation, antibody production, cell respiration and natural growth. Vitamin B-2 is known as *riboflavin,* which helps in alleviating eye fatigue and is important in the prevention and treatment of cataracts. It assists in the metabolism of carbohydrates, fats and proteins, and works in conjunction with vitamin A, which helps maintain the mucous membranes in the digestive tract. Pregnant women must have sufficient amount of riboflavin for the development of the fetus.

Riboflavin deficiency includes symptoms of cracks and sores at the corners of the mouth, eye disorders, inflammation of the mouth and tongue and skin lesions. Other possible deficiency symptoms are dermatitis, dizziness, hair loss, insomnia, light sensitivity, poor digestion, retarded growth and even slow mental responses.[3]

Since riboflavin is involved in energy production, it directly affects your energy level in your sex life. When the B vitamins are insufficient, energy just goes out the door and so does your sex life.

Good food sources of riboflavin are milk, seafood, meat, baby green vegetables, raw nuts and seeds, wheat germ, rice polishings, broccoli, asparagus and soybeans. Good herbal sources are alfalfa and parsley.[4]

Vitamin B-3 is called *niacin* and is needed for proper circulation and healthy skin. It is essential for the nervous

52

system in the metabolism of carbohydrates, fats and proteins, and in the production of hydrochloric acid for proper digestion.

Niacin is involved in the synthesis of sex hormones. It is involved in the normal secretion of bile and stomach fluids. It is used in lowering cholesterol and improving circulation.

When there is a deficiency of niacin, Pellagra (a most irritating skin rash) will develop. Other symptoms of a niacin deficiency include canker sores, dementia, depression diarrhea, dizziness, fatigue, halitosis, headaches, indigestion, insomnia, limb pains, loss of appetite, low blood sugar, muscular weakness, skin eruptions and inflammation.[5]

A word of caution: When taking niacin, you might experience what is called a "niacin flush." A red rash may appear on the skin and a tingling sensation may be felt in the hands and feet.

Good sources of niacin are beef liver, brewer's yeast, broccoli, carrots, cheese, corn flour, dandelion greens, dates, eggs, fish, milk, peanuts, pork, potatoes, tomatoes, wheat germ and whole-wheat products.

Good herbal sources of niacin are alfalfa, parsley and the seeds of burdock, fenugreek, dandelions and sage. These will provide sufficient amounts of niacin.

Vitamin B-6 is called *pyridoxine* and is involved in numerous bodily functions than almost any other single vitamin. It directly affects both our physical and mental health perhaps more than any other of the B vitamins. It is involved in the absorption of fats and protein. Pyridoxine is greatly involved in maintaining sodium and potassium balance and enhances red blood cell formation.

It is now known that B-6 plays a role in cancer immunity and aids in the prevention of arteriosclerosis. Pyridoxine inhibits the formation of a toxic chemical called "homocysteine." Homocysteine attacks the heart muscle and allows the deposition of cholesterol around the heart.[6] New research now shows that if the pituitary is deficient in B-6, there will be a definite loss of the sex drive. B-6 is involved in making epinephrine, which is a neurotransmitter necessary for orgasm.

Symptoms of a B-6 deficiency are neuritis, weakness, irritability, insomnia, anemia, sore tongue and vomiting.[7]

Good sources of B-6 are wheat germ, wheat bran, rice polishings, whole grains, meat, raw nuts, seeds, eggs, honey, molasses, avocados, chicken, fish and spinach.

Vitamin B-5 or *Pantothenic acid* is classified as a B vitamin and is known as an "anti-stress" vitamin. Vitamin B-5 plays a major role in the production of the adrenal hormones and the formation of antibodies, aids in vitamin utilization and assists in the conversion of fats, carbohydrates and proteins into energy.

Pantothenic acid is a stamina enhancer and prevents various kinds of anemia. Vitamin B-5 is needed for normal functioning of the gastrointestinal tract and is known to help relieve depression and anxiety. A deficiency of this vitamin could cause fatigue, headache, nausea and tingling in the hands.

Good food sources of this vitamin are beef, brewer's yeast, eggs, fresh vegetables, kidney, legumes, liver, mushrooms, nuts, pork, royal jelly, saltwater fish, whole-rye flour and whole-wheat flour.

Biotin, another B vitamin, is known as a *micronutrient*. Only a very small amount is needed in human nutrition. If there is a lack of biotin, then depression will take place. Good food sources of biotin may include cereals, vegetables, milk and liver.

PABA is the shortened name for *para-aminobenzoic* acid and is always used in conjunction with folic acid. PABA stimulates the production of good bowel bacteria for the needed folic acid in our diets.

Folic acid, like biotin and PABA, is a member of the B-vitamin family. This wonderful vitamin is most lacking in the American diet. Folic acid is destroyed in the process of cooking. When a person is under stress this vitamin becomes depleted. It is known that miscarriage, fetal malformation and certain anemias can be directly related to a shortage of this most important vitamin.

Good food sources of this vitamin are green leafy vegetables, broccoli, Brussel sprouts, raw nuts, seeds, asparagus, oranges and strawberries.

Choline is needed to make an important brain neurotransmitter, thus it is very important in sexual arousal. A deficiency of this vitamin is linked to high cholesterol, obesity, high blood pressure, heart disease, arteriosclerosis, diabetes and even kidney problems.[8]

Good food sources of this vitamin are egg yoke, meat, poultry, fish, fish roe, soybeans, whole grains, green vegetables, legumes and whole-grain cereals.

Inositol, with PABA and pantothenic acid, is known as the "youth vitamin." Inositol works with choline to help cleanse our livers. It is known to reduce high blood levels of cholesterol. Males need both lecithin and inositol for the sexual fluids that are necessary for reproduction and intercourse.

Good food sources of inositol are whole grains, blackstrap molasses, soybeans, grapefruit, legumes, eggs, raisins and vegetables.

Vitamin B-12 is known as *Cobalamine*. Vitamin B-12 is most necessary to prevent anemia, and it assists folic acid in the regulation and formation of red blood cells. It also helps with the proper utilization of iron. An active form of vitamin B-12 known as "Cyancocobalamin" is required for digestion, absorption of foods, the synthesis of protein and the metabolism of carbohydrates and fats. It is know to prevent nerve damage, maintain fertility and promote normal growth and development by maintaining the fatty sheaths that cover and protects nerve endings. Vitamin B-12 is necessary for the production of acetylcholine, a neurotransmitter that helps with memory and learning abilities.

Vitamin B-12 deficiency can cause an abnormal gait, chronic fatigue, constipation, depression, digestive disorders, hallucinations, headaches, inflammation of the tongue, irritability, palpitations of the heart, pernicious anemia, memory loss and ringing in the ears. This vitamin is so needed by the human body that if there is a deficiency, it can cause great distress and even permanent damage.[9]

Vitamin C

Vitamin C is known as *Ascorbic Acid*. Like the B-vitamins, it too is water soluble, although it is easily lost in cooking. Vitamin C promotes the absorption of vitamins A, B-complex, E, iron and calcium. If there is a deficiency of this vitamin for period of at least four months, scurvy-a disease that attacks the bones and joints-will occur.

This vitamin does affect our sex lives directly through its role in the absorption of iron, the formation of blood cells. In addition, this wonderful vitamin affects the metabolism of the adrenal glands, which stores large amounts of this vitamin. The adrenal glands are known to make a hormone that is involved in stimulation for orgasm. Vitamin C directly helps our joints to remain limber and active, and also stimulates the immune system and helps normalize blood cholesterol levels. One of the major functions of vitamin C is its ability to remove heavy metal minerals and other harmful substances.

Vitamin C is destroyed in the body by smoking, stress, fever, the use of aspirin, antibiotics, cortisone, sulfa drugs, exposure to the pesticide DDT and gasoline fumes.

Signs of vitamin C deficiency are bleeding gums, bruising easily, poor digestion, shortness of breath, nose bleeds, anemia, swollen or painful joints and wounds that do not heal readily.

Good food sources of vitamin C are strawberries, tomatoes, mangos, Brussels sprouts, avocados, citrus fruits, asparagus, cantaloupe and green vegetables.[10]

Vitamin D

Vitamin D is a fat-soluble vitamin and is required for the absorption and utilization of calcium and phosphorus by the intestinal tract. Vitamin D protects against muscle weakness and is directly involved in the regulation of the heart beat. Calcium with vitamin D helps prevent osteoporosis and hypocalcemia, it enhances immunity necessary for good thyroid function.[11]

When there is a deficiency of vitamin D, this will cause rickets in children and osteomalacia, a similar disorder found in adults. Lesser deficiencies will bring out loss of appetite, a burning sensation in the mouth and throat, diarrhea, insomnia, visual problems and even weight loss.

A word of caution: Do not take vitamin D without calcium being present. Toxicity can result if an individual takes over 65,000 international units over a period of time.

Vitamin E

Vitamin E is a most wonderful vitamin since it works as an antioxidant that is most important in the prevention of cancer and cardiovascular disease. It is known to improve circulation and is needed for tissue repair. It has been used successfully in treating premenstrual syndrome and fibrocystic disease of the breast. This glorious vitamin helps reduce high blood pressure, aids in preventing cataracts, improves athletic performance and relaxes leg cramps.[12]

Since vitamin E is an antioxidant, it prevents cell damage by inhibiting the oxidation of lipids (fats) and the formation of free floating radicals. It aids in the utilization of vitamin A and helps protect it by preventing destruction of it from oxidation. Many scientists believe that it helps prevent the aging process.

Vitamin E is necessary for fertility in both men and women. A shortage of this vitamin may cause menstrual problems, neuromuscular impairment, shortened red blood cell life span, miscarriage and uterine degeneration. It is now known that low levels of vitamin E have been linked to bowel cancer and breast cancer.[13]

Good food sources of vitamin E are cold-pressed vegetable oils, dark green leafy vegetables, legumes, nuts, seeds and whole grains. Varied amounts of vitamin E may be found in brown rice, cornmeal, dulse, eggs, kelp, milk, oatmeal, soybeans, sweet potatoes, watercress, wheat and wheat germ. Several good herbs that contain E are alfalfa, bladderwrack, dandelion, dong guai, flaxseed, nettle oat straw, raspberry leaf and rose hips.[14]

Do not exceed more than 1,200 I.U. of vitamin E per day. Excessive amounts of vitamin E have been known to cause rapid heart beat.

Vitamin F-Essential Fatty Acids

Vitamin F, or *Essential Fatty Acids,* have often been forgotten by many seeking to improve their health, but this is not a good thing to do. The essential fatty acids consists of linoleic, linolenic, and arachidonic acids (unsaturated fatty acids), but vitamin F is not made by the human body.

Vitamin F is most important for your sex life since it is needed by the thyroid gland, adrenal glands and prostate as well as to manufacture prostaglandins—a group of chemical substances that work synergistically with hormones.

This vitamin encourages calcium absorption, slows cholesterol build up, regulates blood coagulation, aids in forming membranes, causes beautiful shiny hair and moistens the skin.[15]

If this vitamin is not sufficiently present in the diet it will cause diarrhea, weight loss, varicose veins, brittle hair, dandruff, skin disorders, problems with fat metabolism and a lower immune system.

Good food sources of this vitamin F are raw nuts and seeds, whole grains, wheat germ, whole milk and vegetable oils.

We should find our vitamins in the foods that we eat. Of course, this is going to take planning and time in preparation of food. Although natural vitamins are best, vitamin supplements should be taken if, for some good reason, we know that we are not getting what our body truly needs. Natural vitamins are more readily digestible and will work more effectively in our bodies. Of course, there is much disagreement about this when compared to taking synthetic vitamins.

If you truly want to improve your sex life, eat a most balanced healthy diet. Remember there is no easy road to good health. Good food coupled with minerals, vitamins and exercise will revolutionize your sex life. You will see your body respond by giving you radiant health.

Chapter 6

Glorious Nutrients for a Better Sex Life

Nutrients in our daily diet are an important part of good nutrition, which can lead to good sex. We've looked at minerals and vitamins, but let's look at other natural substances that will ensure us a healthy life.

Ginkgo Biloba

Many woman suffer from premenstrual syndrome, which begins a week or two before menstruation. It is believed that at one time or another 90 percent of all women will suffer premenstrual syndrome. One of the big problems many women incur during menstruation is the problem of water retention, swollen and tender breasts, and many other numerous symptoms. What to do? There is help in the wonderful herb called "Ginkgo Biloba."

Many women in the United States will take water pills and laxatives to rid their bodies of fluid. This is very wrong! Taking these drugs will actually reduce the amount of potassium in your body. The effects of laxatives are only temporary, and the side effects of taking them are enormous. You actually set yourself up for what is known as "lazy bowel syndrome." The natural rhythm of the bowel is quenched and constipation becomes a way of life. Another problem that occurs with those women who repeatedly take laxatives is that they become psychologically addicted to them.

There is now proof that Ginkgo Biloba may reduce water retention during and prior to menstruation. Researchers at Henri Mondor Hospital in Creteil, France, report in the September 25, 1986 issue of *La Presse Medicale* that Ginkgo actually reduced water retention substantially in those women given 160 milligrams and 200 milligrams on a daily basis. Some women never suffered from water retention again. Many had definite improvement in the various controlled groups.[1]

Other women who had suffered from severe water retention were given larger dosages of Ginkgo as much as 200 to 300 milligrams. These women lost as much as four to ten pounds in four to five days.[2] The final conclusions were that Ginkgo Biloba was most effective against congestive symptoms of PMS, particularly breast discomfort and irritability.[3]

Impotence

There are certain men who at times experience the inability to have or to maintain an erection. Impotence is experienced occasionally by many men, but when it develops into a chronic condition, it then becomes a real problem. It is estimated that 30 million men in the United States suffer from it, but only one-tenth will ever seek medical advice.[4] Many men assume that this problem is hopeless. Others are just to embarrassed to talk about it with their doctors, and they assume it is an unnatural weakness.

In the majority of men, impotence is usually caused by psychological factors. Impotence may be short term caused by stress or fatigue or, longstanding, caused by anxiety and guilt that might have originated in early childhood. Impotence may be a symptom of depression.[5]

It is estimated that 10 percent of impotence is caused by a physical disorder (including diabetes mellitus or hormonal imbalance) or by a neurological disorder (such as spinal cord damage or chronic alcohol abuse). Various antipsychotics, antidepressants, antihypertensive and diuretics will cause impotence. As men get older, impotence becomes more likely. Undoubtedly this is due to altered circulation or less often, lowered levels of the male sex hormone testosterone.[6]

We do know that there are numerous causes of male impotence in men of all ages. Most of these are physical in origin caused by problems with blood vessels or some kind of disorder of their nervous system. Usually the problem is with the circulatory system or possible nerve damage.

High blood pressure, diminished testosterone levels and side effects of medication taken for other conditions all contribute to this problem of impotence. It is interesting to note that men who have intense physical jobs are most likely to experience problems and injuries. The most common cause of impotence is the blockage of blood to the male sex organ.

Recent studies have shown that Ginkgo Biloba improve circulation to all blood vessels. Recent experiments have shown that Ginkgo can help prevent impotence due to restriction in the blood vessels of the penis.[7] Ginkgo shows promise as a treatment for sexual problems related to the usage of prescribed anti-depressant drugs such as Prozac and Zoloft.[8]

Since the propensity of Ginkgo is dilation of the blood vessels, it makes good sense to use this marvelous herb if there is difficulty in obtaining an erection. Since an erection requires not only arousal but the action of both the nervous and circulatory systems, Ginkgo directly helps to dilate blood vessels. Consequently there is good reason to use Ginkgo when erectile problems exist.

There is relatively little research about the usage of Ginkgo for erectile problems. Common sense and the long use of Ginkgo in Asian medicine indicate that this herb is beneficial for aiding in male potency problems.

I would recommend that men who have problems with erections and women who have problems with PMS take Ginkgo Biloba for the course of several months. Take note whether the symptoms are easing or not. It is most possible that Ginkgo will be a good natural treatment.

Aloe Vera

There is so much talk about Aloe Vera but much of it is pure folklore. *Aloe barbadensis* is the scientific name for this plant. It is thick-leaved, spiny-edged succulent plant from which we may obtain the juice. Aloe Vera is even mentioned in the Bible and is known for its healing properties. This wonderful herb may be used internally and externally. It acts as a mild tonic for the body.

Aloe Vera juice is of the utmost value in cleansing and soothing the internal organs especially the stomach, pancreas, liver, kidneys, lungs, glands and has the effect of stimulating the uterus. Many people have a tingling and warm sensation in their internal organs as the body undergoes a deep cleansing while taking the aloe vera juice.

It is known that aloe vera contains as many as 75 biologically active ingredients including several B vitamins, choline and vitamin C. At the same time calcium, chlorine, manganese, potassium, sodium and natural sulphur may be found in aloe vera.[9]

In addition to the many vitamins in aloe vera there are 18 amino acids, many plant sugars, natural "antibiotics," which are called anthra quimones, that cleanse and stop itching and reducing inflammation.[10] Aloe vera has at least five different enzymes. This wonderful herb contains a potent fungicide that has proven most effective against athlete's feet and other stubborn fungus infections.[11]

Aloe vera may be used on the skin for rashes or inflammation. It has a wonderful soothing effect. The juice of aloe may be even used as a douche for vaginitis. It has a most wonderful effect on colitis when used as an enema.

Chlorella

There is on the market today a product called "Chlorella." Chlorella is an edible microalga grown under strict supervision in large tanks in order to create one of the most wonderful products known to humankind. Chlorella is full of DNA and RNA and other beneficial nutrients.

As man gets older, the production in the human body of RNA and DNA decreases with age, resulting in lower vitality and other signs of aging. It is recommended to take Chlorella three times a day to counteract the aging process. Chlorella is a most excellent source of chlorophyll, nature's foremost cleanser and detoxifier. It also is excellent as a source to build up one's blood and it is an excellent source of B-12.

Chlorella is one of the finest supplements in our day to restore or enhance the reproductive system. This wonderful microalga cleanses, strengthens and builds up every gland, organ and tissue in the human body. Consequently, it is most beneficial for the sex glands since they become enhanced with the usage of chlorella. Not only this, but chlorella improves bowel elimination by feeding the bowel beneficial flora and improves the peristaltic motion.

Chlorella purifies the liver and strengthens liver function. The Japanese use chlorella in the treatment of cirrhosis of the liver. It also helps the body to eliminate toxic metals assisting as a cleanser and detoxifier.

Cell repair through the body is stimulated and aided by the nucleic factors found in chlorella. It strengthens the immune system and helps protect against debilitating illness and disease.[12] It affects the sexual glands by strengthening them through nucleic factors found in the alga.

Chlorella tends to keep the body free of debilitating, energy-sapping substances and conditions. As a result of this, we are more readily able to enjoy our sexuality with our partner.

Garlic

Garlic has always been considered a total body tonic. Alliin, a sulfur-containing amino acid, is one of the active ingredients found in garlic. It converts to allicin, which gives garlic its distinctive odor. Garlic acts as an antibiotic, antibacterial, antifungal agent.[13] Garlic is known to reduce blood cholesterol level as well as triglyceride level. It helps against narrowing of the arteries, and it acts as a blood thinner and an excellent antioxidant. It helps the body to eliminate toxic metals and even lowers blood pressure. It is believed to help protect against certain types of cancer.

It is a known fact that men and women who chew garlic in Bulgaria live to be beyond one hundred years of age. Many of these people are still sexually active even at the age of one hundred and beyond. Garlic is a contributing factor to their sex lives.

If you should find the odor of garlic offensive, you can buy brands that don't have an odor. Odorless garlic works just as well as regular garlic.

Bee Pollen

The effects of taking honeybee pollen has long been known to stimulate the sexual system. Pollen is about 20 percent protein and is quite rich in fatty acids and carbohydrates. It has natural steroids, which are believed to stimulate the sex glands.

Research has been done in Russia that supports the fact that pollen actually benefited the endocrine system. The Russians have also found that taking bee pollen shortened the recovery time of surgery in both men and women. Both German and Swedish scientists have found a hormone in pollen that does stimulate the sex glands.[14]

Herbal Teas

Perhaps the best way to take herbs is by making a tea out of them. Herbal teas are milder, safer and have fewer side effects or drugs. Remember that herbs are food and not manmade medicines. Consequently, they take a little longer to work and have far fewer adverse effects. If you should have a side effect from taking an herb, stop taking it and try another that may have similar properties.

When making a tea you may use the roots and bark which are called a "decoction." When leaves or blossoms are used this is called an "infusion." It is now possible not only to buy the raw materials from the health food shop, but many grocery stores are now selling them. If you buy the herb in capsule form you may break the capsule, open it and use it in the making of your tea.

Get the directions from a good book on herbs from your local health food store. These numerous new books will give great detail on how to make your teas. They also will recommend certain herbs for various ailments that you might be experiencing. It is an investment in your health that you will treasure all of your life.

God has provided in nature His very own nutrients and herbs that can help in overcoming sexual problems. These nutrients and herbs will actually heal, cleanse and invigorate various glands and organs of the body. It may take as long as two or three months for them to become effective but keep on taking them. You will see results and even an improvement in your overall health.

Chapter 7

Your Glands and Good Sex

The health of our endocrine system determines if our sex life is good. The endocrine glands create an internal energy within the human body that is needed for good sex. If the health of an individual is poor, then he lacks energy for anything, much less sex.

If other glands in the body are not functioning properly, this will cause a lack of energy, which may be a result of hypothyroidism (low thyroid function) or hypoglycemia (low blood sugar) due to malfunctioning of the Islets of Langerhans. In my home state of Minnesota, our soil is almost depleted of selenium, which is so needed for proper immune function. Low thyroid functioning is not uncommon in the Northern States since the soil is almost depleted of many needed minerals for our diet.

When married couples engage in sexual intercourse, hormone changes cause them to have an appearance of youthfulness. Our entire glandular system is stimulated when we engage in sexual activity. Good marital sex in marriage encourages better self-esteem and more self-confidence.

We cannot over stress the importance of the endocrine system and its role in sexual activity. The endocrine glands are a network of ductless glands and other structures that elaborate and secret their hormones directly into the bloodstream. The result of this is the direct targeting of specific glands. Glands of the endocrine system include the thyroid and the parathyroid, the anterior and posterior pituitary, the pancreas, the suprarenal glands, ovaries and the testes. The pineal gland is also considered an endocrine gland since it is a ductless gland. We are not totally aware of the function of the pineal gland.[1]

The endocrine system functions by releasing chemical messengers from specific glands. These chemical messengers are hormones that enter the bloodstream and are designed to stimulate certain kinds of activity for various tissues. Endocrine glands are able to initiate nerve impulses just as nerves are able to initiate or inhibit hormone release.

It is essential to avoid stress as much as possible. I am aware that this sounds rather ludicrous, but stress does hinder and weaken glandular function. Stress first attacks the weaker glands and, as time goes on, it affects all glandular activity. We need to learn to handle our problems better and manage stress appropriately.

It is the glands of our bodies that give us enjoyment and pleasure, so it behooves us to get enough exercise and sufficient rest so that they will function at peak levels. In many ways, we are as old as we feel.

Basically there are three types of hormones produced by the endocrine system. These are polypeptide hormones, steroid hormones and prostaglandins.[2]

Polypeptide hormones act as a type of "messenger hormone." These hormones trigger a release of other hormones such as estrogen, testosterone and progesterone. These are all sexual hormones so very necessary for normal functioning of both male and female organs. They also function in the brain as neurotransmitters (nerve transmitters).[3] Hormones are very powerful as they affect certain tissues for which God designed them. They have the propensity to change the metabolism of every tissue found within the body. They work in conjunction with other hormones causing the release of additional hormones.[4]

Let's take a good look at the glands of the endocrine system and their function.

Pituitary Gland: The pituitary gland is often referred to as the master gland and is the most important of the endocrine glands. This gland regulates and controls the activities of the other glands of the endocrine system. It also assists in many other body processes.[5] It is found in the base of the brain and assists in growth, sexual development and fertility.[6]

Thyroid Gland: The thyroid gland is an important organ of the endocrine system. The thyroid gland is situated in the front of the neck, just below the larynx. The thyroid gland consists of two lobes, one on either side of the trachea (wind pipe), joined by a narrower portion of tissue known as the isthmus.[7] The thyroid controls the metabolism of the entire body and regulates energy production and oxygen. It also assists in regulating blood calcium.[8]

Pineal Gland: The pineal gland is a tiny, cone-shaped body within the brain. It appears that the only function of the pineal gland is the secretion of melatonin. Melatonin is a hormone necessary for good sleep.9 It is possible that the pineal gland effects ovarian secretion, menstrual cycle and possibly stimulates the adrenals to produce the sex hormone aldosterone.[10]

Parathyroid Glands: The parathyroid glands consist of two pairs of oval, pea-sized glands located adjacent to the two lobes of the thyroid gland in the neck. These glands produce the parathyroid hormone that helps control the level of calcium in the blood. These glands are constantly regulating hormone levels since even a small variation from normal can impair muscle and nerve function.[11]

Adrenal Glands: The adrenal glands are a pair of endocrine glands that secrete hormones directly into the bloodstream. They are small and triangular and sit on top of the kidneys. They are involved with carbohydrate metabolism, healing, heart rate, blood pressure, blood sugar, water and electrolyte recovery. They are most important in the formation of male and female hormones.[12]

Prostate Gland: The prostate gland is a solid, chestnut-shaped organ surrounding the first part of the urethra in the male. The prostate gland is situated immediately under the bladder and in front of the rectum.[13] The prostate produces fluid to protect the male sperm.

Islets of Langerhans: The Islets of Langerhans are endocrine cells located in the pancreas. They secrete digestive enzymes into a network of ducts that meet to form the main pancreatic duct.[14]

Thymus Gland: The thymus gland is part of the immune system. It is situated in the upper part of the chest, behind the breast bone and consists of two lobes that join in front of the trachea. It aids the immune system by producing special killer cells called "T-cells."[15]

Ovaries: The ovaries consist of a pair of almond-shaped glands situated on either side of the uterus just below the opening of the fallopian tube. Each ovary is about 1.25 inch (30 mm) long and 0.75 inches (20 mm) wide and contains numerous cavities called "follicles" in which egg cells develop. In addition to producing eggs, they also produce hormones such as estrogen and progesterone.[16]

Testes: The testes are located in the male pelvic area. They are in the male scrotum and produce sperm and the male sex hormone testosterone.[17]

Hypothalamus: The hypothalamus is about the size of a cherry, situated behind the eyes and beneath another brain region called the thalamus. The hypothalamus also aids in the coordination of the function of the nervous and endocrine (hormonal) systems of the entire body. The hypothalamus indirectly controls many of the endocrine glands including the pituitary, thyroid, adrenal cortex and gonads.[18]

We hear a lot of talk about steroid hormones. These hormones are fatty-based substances with a cholesterol type nucleus, such as the hormones produced and secreted from the adrenal cortex, ovaries and testicles. Steroids aid in carbohydrate, fat and protein metabolism. They also assist the body in handling stress and help prevent certain kinds of infections. They have been misused in the past by weight lifters and other athletes wanting to add muscle mass on their bodies. Excessive use of steroids is dangerous and may even cause cancer.

We need to mention the importance of the prostaglandins. These are made from fatty acids and are not hormones. They are not produced in the endocrine system but in certain areas of the body where local cells utilize them. They aid in raising or lowering blood pressure and help in stimulating the production of steroids.[19]

When there is a chemical imbalance of the glands, there may be excessive strain on the glands and all kinds of physical problems may ensure as a result. To have good sex, your glands need to be healthy.

From Puberty to Adulthood

For a moment let us consider the subject of puberty both in males and females. Puberty is that time in the life of an adolescent when the secondary sexual characteristics develop and the sexual organs mature, allowing reproduction to become possible. The term puberty is the word that we use for the physical changes that underlie the emotional development of adolescence. Puberty usually occurs between the ages of 10 and 15 in both of the sexes. This comes about by the initiation of the pituitary gland producing hormones known as *gonadotropins*. These will stimulate the ovaries to produce the secretion of estrogen hormones and the testes to increase the secretion of testosterone. Puberty is accompanied by a significant growth spurt and increase of body weight.

The first sign of puberty in girls is usually breast growth, which usually occurs around the age of eleven. In about one-third of the girls, pubic hair appears first. Menstruation comes after the evidence of pubic hair and breast growth. Other secondary sexual characteristics, such as a wider pelvis and fat distribution develop during this time of puberty. When the menstrual cycle is regular, puberty is considered to have finished.

Puberty in boys is heralded by a sudden increase of the rate of the growth of the testicles and scrotum, followed by the growth of facial hair and pubic hair. The sexual organs begin to grow around the age of thirteen and reach adult size about two years later. Again there are variations of development due to the release of testosterone. The body's increased secretion of testosterone stimulates the production of sperm and increases the size of the seminal vesicles. At the same time the prostate gland begins to enlarge. The facial hair, chest and abdominal hair appear during this time. The larynx enlarges and the vocal cords become longer and thicker. As a result of this, the voice starts to become deeper.[20]

As adolescents mature into adulthood, the diet and lifestyle they lead when younger will reflect in the later years. Good eating habits, exercise and a healthy outlook on life will prepare their bodies and minds for a physical relationship with their future mates and, eventually, parenthood.

DHEA and Melatonin: Good or Bad?

God has given us several wonderful hormones that directly effect every area of our lives. No other hormones have received so much publicity as DHEA and Melatonin—the anti-aging hormones. These two hormones are now available in health food stores, K-Mart, Target and just about everywhere. But what is the real truth about DHEA and Melatonin?

DHEA, "dehydroepiandrosterone," comes from the adrenal glands and melatonin comes from the pineal gland. It is probably best to look at each of these individually.

It is known that DHEA improves memory, reduces the risk of heart attack, helps with fat loss and improves immune function. It is very true that DHEA is the most abundant steroid hormone in the human body. It is synthesized in the range of 25 to 30 mg daily. The second most abundant is cortisol, which is synthesized at a rate of about 10 to 290 mg produced everyday. If the person is under stress then cortisol output is higher.[21]

The body produces a substantial amount of DHEA since it acts as an inhibitor over cortisol action by binding to its receptors.[22] DHEA represents another feedback control mechanism to cause a greater action of eicosanoids by inhibiting the inhibitor (cortisol) of eicosanoids synthesis.[23] Eicosanoids are very powerful autocrine hormones.

Many authorities have reported low levels of DHEA in diabetes, coronary artery disease, various cancers, obesity, lupus erythematosus, hypertension, AIDS, viral infections, Alzheimer's disease, and multiple sclerosis.[24] It should be noted that DHEA deficiency is a reflection of the maladaptation in all of these stress-related illnesses.

It has been noted that increased testosterone and DHEA are associated with lower insulin levels in men but in women increased levels of testosterone and DHEA are related to hyperinsulinemia and insulin resistance.[25]

DHEA levels are decreased when patients are given cortisol and prednisone. In addition to this, in a group of older men and women from 77 to 79 years of age, the higher functioning subjects all had higher levels of DHEA and many fewer psychiatric symptoms.[26]

DHEA modulates diabetes, obesity, carcinogenesis, tumor growth, stress, pregnancy, hypertension, collagen and skin integrity, fatigue, depression, memory and immune response.[27] In male diabetics, DHEA does help in normal erections. Since many male diabetes do have problems in that area, it is very important to have the blood checked for DHEA levels.

DHEA's major role is as a homeostatic mechanism in the basic stress reaction. When one is stressed, too much cortisol is released to raise blood sugar levels. Then there is a release of glycogen from the liver, which is broken down into glucose and gently released into the bloodstream. This in turn releases insulin for the functioning of burning excess glucose. If there is a gradual maladaptation in the glucose-insulin regulatory mechanism, this may be the first stage of decreased DHEA. DHEA has an antiviral effect on the body, but if there is an abnormal modulation of the homeostatic insulin-glucose effects, the immune system is directly affected.

Caffeine, nicotine and sugar are dangerous because all of them induce a stress reaction and do raise blood sugar levels. This results in elevated blood sugar levels, which in turn slows down the production of DHEA.

DHEA is so essential to the diabetic person. Very early in the course of diabetes, there is a loss of sensitivity to insulin. DHEA is almost certainly the choice of treatment in the very early stages of diabetes, especially adult-onset diabetes, Type O. Anyone diagnosed with diabetes must reduce the amount of calories they take in, increase their exercise and reduce the amount of stress. It has been noted that with the introduction of DHEA that many symptoms of diabetes disappeared.

Before taking DHEA on your own, it is best that your physician do blood work to determine your DHEA level. If the DHEA blood level is below 550 ng/dL in a woman or below 750 ng/dL in a man, then natural stimulation of the body should be taken into consideration. If this is not done, then supplementation with DHEA should be considered.[28] It is my personal opinion that DHEA is far safer than many diabetic drugs.

Many diabetic people are overweight and need to lose substantial amounts of weight to regain overall good health. DHEA serves to enhance fat metabolism and to assist in weight reduction in patients who are obese. Research has shown that dogs put on DHEA along with a high fiber content lost 65.7 percent of their excess body weight.[29] In obese men, there was a 31 percent loss of body fat in the men treated with DHEA. It should be noted that there was no change in body weight but body fat was down by 31 percent. It is thought that DHEA curbs hunger. The latest research on DHEA in obesity reveals that weight loss leads to insulin reduction and a 125 percent increase in DHEA in men.[30]

Melatonin

God has created this wonderful hormone to give us sound sleep and keep us youthful. Melatonin is produced by the pineal gland, and it is most abundant in young people but decreases as people get older. It is available as a non-prescription supplement in capsule form.

Melatonin is stimulated by darkness, but the secretion does stop during the daylight. It is known to induce sleep, regulate metabolic rate, increases longevity, protects from free radical damage and will enhance the immune system.

It is now known that low levels of this hormone are implicated in breast cancer, melanoma, dysfunction and depression. Melatonin does cross barriers to enter cells and is a non-toxic hormone. It is known to inhibit secretion of estrogen and slows breast, cervical and skin cancer development.[31] It is a most potent anti-aging hormone which, when taken on a regular basis, can have dramatic effects. Production of this hormone can be lowered by electromagnetic fields, strong light at night while sleeping, alcohol consumption, aging, heart medications such as betablockers and diuretics.[32]

Melatonin is excellent for the relieve of insomnia, depression, SAD and even jet lag. It does strengthen the immune system when the body is under stress. It is known to protect against free radical damage, decreases pain and can be used to slow the progression of Alzheimer's disease. In addition to this, it protects against various cancers and will aid in the prevention of premature aging.

This hormone should not be taken if you are under forty years of age because your body is making enough melatonin at this time. It should be taken about a half-hour before bedtime and in small doses. This hormone must not be used by people with Hodgkin's disease, Lymphoma or multiple myeloma as there can be some side effects.[33]

When there are low levels of melatonin, the immune system begins to shut down. At the same time they signal the endocrine system to produce fewer sex hormones. If this should occur lower levels of sex hormones in turn may lead to the atrophy of sexual organs in both men and women, a lack of interest in sex and definite poor sexual performance.

It has been demonstrated in rats that by giving them larger doses of melatonin that their sexual organs were regenerated. Therefore, one can conclude it is very possible that the same thing could happen with human beings. Melatonin may actually cause regeneration and rejuvenation, making them comparable to those of younger humans. This is still in the laboratory-study stage and has not been proven at this time. Do not take large amounts of melatonin thinking that your sex life will be totally restored since it could be most harmful.

A healthy glandular system is vital to your body *and* your marriage. Learn to take good care of yourself.

Chapter 8

Male Sexual Problems
and the Prostate

If you are a man somewhere over the age of fifty, you need to know about your prostate gland. Have you been having frequent urination, especially at night? This problem may not be with your bladder but with your prostate gland. Especially if you're making frequent trips to the bathroom at night, this could be a disorder of your prostate.

Every year in the United States about 40,000 men will die of prostate cancer. This terrible disease is on the increase among the men of this country. Most men don't know what the function of the prostate is and where it is located.

This walnut-sized organ is located next to the bladder and surrounds the urethra. The urethra is the canal through which the urine passes out of the body. The prostate gland produces the liquid that acts as a vehicle for the sperm cells which, during intercourse, are secreted into the vagina. The purpose of this is the fertilization of the female's egg, the end result being reproduction. Without this little gland, the male will become sterile.

A normal prostate gland empties its fluid into the urethra at the moment of orgasm. When the prostate is abnormal in size, it puts pressure on the urethra, thus increasing the time to empty the bladder. As the prostate enlarges, the greater the pressure and the more difficult it becomes to totally empty the bladder.[1]

If you are having a hard time with your prostate gland, you may be experiencing prostatitis, which is an inflammation of the prostate. Here are a few warning signs.

With prostatitis there is always a feeling of congestion and discomfort in the pubic area.[2] The bladder always feels as though it is full, with the necessity of making frequent trips to the bathroom especially during the night hours. On occasions it will become most difficult to avoid; rarely will there be any passage of urine.

The need to urinate during the night hours is most distressing. It interrupts your sleep. Then there is the problem of waste residue collecting in the bladder, but some release may be possible. This condition can become serious if the urethra becomes blocked. The probability of uremic poisoning arises when the bladder becomes overloaded with fluid.[3] If the waste is not discharged it can flood the kidneys, presenting a most serious danger of poisoning to the entire system.

Understand that prostate problems do not just go away and it is most advisable to see a physician as soon as possible. There is the possibility that the ailing prostate will become so enlarged it will constrict the urethra and completely block the flow of urine. This condition is extremely painful and could be fatal if not treated at once.

Here is a list of warning signals that might indicate problems with the prostate.

1. Pain in the lower back.
2. The presence of blood in the urine or in the seminal excretion.

3. Frequent erections without any prior stimulation.

4. Pain during the release of the seminal fluid.

5. Erectile problems (impotence and/or premature ejaculation).

6. A persistent sense of fullness in the bowels and difficult in elimination of waste.

7. Difficulties either in starting the urine stream or the inability to stop the flow of urine could mean a loss of control.

Men over fifty years of age should have their prostate gland checked at least once a year. This is a precaution that could assist in the prevention of serious health problems.

The aging process affects men in other ways than a woman who has under gone menopause. Very few men experience a sudden loss of reproductive ability comparable with that in a women. The aging process does bring noticeable changes to the male sex organs. Sperm production also declines with age, but there are cases of men in their nineties who were still able to father children. It is very certain in many cases that the aging process will bring on impotence but often times the cause is psychological and not physical.

About the age of sixty however, the general aging process results in noticeable changes to the male sex organs.[4] There maybe hardening of blood vessels leading to the erectile tissue in the penis making it very difficult to obtain an erection. The scrotal tissue sags and eventually will even wrinkle. The testes shrink and lose firmness and their elevation on excitement is greatly reduced.

There will come a diminished production of sperm as the result of thickening and degeneration of the seminiferous tubules. The prostate gland often times enlarges, and its contractions during orgasm become much weaker making intercourse less pleasurable.

In the average male, production of the sex hormone testosterone, peaks in early adulthood and then begins to decline in old age. At around the age of sixty when the rate of decline slows down, the amount produced is very similar to that of a nine- or ten-year-old boy. It is interesting to note that production usually remains sufficient for sexual activity to continue into extreme old age.

The ability to enjoy sex can continue well into old age, particularly if the couple makes a concerted effort to understand and respond to the various changes that age brings to the natural pattern of sexual response.[5] Often times older couples give up intercourse because they mistakenly interpret body changes as signs of future impotence. Lovemaking may have to become a more leisurely affair for older couple. There are great benefits of maintaining the physical side of sex as the couple gets older.

If prostate health is good, older men can enjoy sexual intercourse just as much as when they were younger. Older men generally need a longer period of time before an erection occurs; when they achieve an erection it usually takes minutes rather than seconds for it to happen. Once an erection is achieved, however, they have the advantage of being able to maintain it for a much longer time than when they were younger. Older men are able to control their ejaculatory ability for a longer time, which allows the intercourse to be extended for a longer period of time.

Although orgasm is reached more slowly by older men, orgasm itself is completed more rapidly. Indeed, orgasmic contractions are not as strong, the force of ejaculation is reduced, and the seminal fluid is thinner and substantially reduced in volume.[6]

Common Prostate Problems

Acute prostatitis is an inflammation of the prostate coupled with a bacterial infection.[7] The symptoms may include fever, chills and painful urination with possible pain in the lower back and between the legs. When this occurs it makes sexual intercourse virtually impossible.

Chronic prostatitis is an infection that comes and goes. Symptoms of this disease are the same as the acute form but may be milder. Massaging the prostate has proven beneficial in releasing the blocked fluids.

Benign prostatic hypertrophy (BPH) is an enlargement of the prostate gland. This disease is related to small non-cancerous tumors that grow inside the prostate.[8]

Prostate cancer is a malignant growth arising in the outer zone of the prostate. Today this disease claims one-third of the newly diagnosed cancers among men in this country. If the disease is not diagnosed early it may spread to other organs and death will occur. When symptoms do appear they are similar to those of BPH. BPH is related to the changing hormone level as one ages.

A urologist—a specialist in disorders of the urinary system—understands these problems.

The best way to protect yourself against disease of the prostate is to have a yearly examination as previously mentioned. If symptoms occur go to your health care practitioner as soon as possible, it could save your life.

Therapy

Paramount to dealing with disease of the prostate and prevention, is an adequate intake and absorption of the mineral zinc. Zinc is probably so successful in the treatment of this disease of the prostate because it is involved with many aspects of hormonal metabolism. . This mineral is necessary for sperm formation and function, sexual health and other reproductive hormone systems. For men, zinc may be considered the key, not only to good prostate health, but the key to a good sex life.

The prostate accumulates very high levels of zinc-about ten times more than any other organ of the body. When benign hypertrophy is existent there is a deficiency of zinc.

Zinc has a unique influence on sperm as sperm must swim to the woman's fallopian tubes so penetration of the egg will take place for fertilization.

Zinc may be found in brewer's yeast, nuts, eggs, rice bran, onions, chicken, beans, peas, lentils, wheat germ and wheat bran. Be cautious about the amount of eggs and chicken that you eat since they tend to be high in cholesterol. Try to find as many other sources of food as possible so you receive the zinc you need. Zinc is also available at the health food stores and pharmacies. It is believed that thirty-five milligrams per day of zinc will build up resistance to prostate disorders and even relieve the symptoms it produces.

Zinc actually acts as a catalyst in many biological reactions to nourish and even rejuvenate the prostate. Amino acids and nutrients are brought together by the zinc to aid in the repair of delicate tissues and tubules of the prostate to keep it in a youthful condition. Since zinc plays a role in carbohydrate metabolism, the energy source is build into the prostate to keep it alive, healthy and young.[9]

Certainly as a child you ate pumpkin seeds. These wonderful seeds are full of vitamins and minerals and are an excellent source of vegetable protein. These tasty seeds are a source of essential fatty acids, which the prostate readily absorbs.

Essential fatty acids are well known for preserving the health, virility and even the potency for the prostate.[10] These concentrated nutrients in pumpkin seeds work in conjunction with zinc to keep the delicate tubules, cells and tissues in smooth working order. These nutrients actually enter right into the prostatic fluid maintaining the vigor, strength and fitness of the gland. Linoleic acid, linolenic acid and arachidonic acid help keep the heart healthy and make a positive difference to your prostate.

If you don't like eating pumpkin seeds, then buy pumpkin seed capsules at the local health food store. Pumpkin seeds and oil work like a miracle drug in prostate rejuvenation. Sunflower seed oil, wheat germ oil, soybean oil and sesame seed oil are full of Essential Fatty Acids. Walnuts, Brazil nuts, pine nuts, peanuts, pecans and almonds help the prostate to remain healthy.

Let us not forget the great benefits that come from garlic. Garlic is a powerful store house of natural antibiotics that help insulate the prostate from infection and bacteria. According to Professor Gurwitch, a European electrobologist, garlic releases an ultraviolet radiation called mitogenetic radiations.[11] These rays have the ability of stimulating cell growth and activity of the prostate. Garlic appears to have a natural antibiotic property that shields the prostate against parasitic infection. Garlic has the ability to assist in repair and reconstruct weakened glandular tissues so that the organ will remain healthy.

Garlic is full of allicin, which has the propensity to cleanse away decomposed bacteria. Garlic helps prevent prostate infection since it has the ability to destroy certain strains of bacteria. Garlic possess a powerful penetrative force unlike many other herbs.[12] Dr. Gurwitch's research indicates that garlic is able to uproot and discharge infections and bacteria, which allow the prostate to regenerate itself. Cut up a few cloves of garlic and put them in a salad with pumpkin seeds. Try a tablespoon of sesame seeds in your salad dressing and you will have a powerful tonic for the prostate.

Herbs That Boost Sexual Ability

Though herbal cures are rarely backed with detail research in traditional medicine, there is good evidence that some herbs actually help with sexual performance. Please be advised that it takes several weeks before these herbs to work. As with any program, be sure to consult your doctor before starting an herbal program. If you are taking prescribed drugs, they could have a drug interaction.

Ginkgo Biloba: Ginkgo is one of the most studied of all herbs. It improves blood flow throughout the body by relaxing the arteries. This herb can aid men with erectile problems caused by vascular disease.

In 1989, a study was done in Germany with a group of men-half of which were taking 60 milligrams (mg) a day of this herb. After six months, the results were those men who took the herb regained their ability to have erections.[13] Another study that was presented to the national urology conference of 1998 found that men who took ginkgo had slightly more rigid overnight erections than men who had not taken the herb.

Ginkgo is considered safe in doses up to 240 mg a day. Many doctors recommend men desiring to take this herb should begin with 80 mg. There is a note of caution: "There have been some rare cases of complications associated with the combined use of ginkgo and aspirin, so it's especially important to check with the doctor if you take aspirin regularly," says Tieraona Low Dog, M.L., director of the New Mexico School of Herbal Medicine and Research in Albuquerque, New Mexico.[14]

Ginseng: This most wonderful herb contains ginsenosides, compounds that researchers believe can improve proness by increasing hormone levels. "Ginseng encourages the body to make more testosterone, and it has been shown to increase sperm production," says Dr. Low Dog.[15]

It is important to check the label for the designation "Panax." This means that the herb is of American or oriental source. Most ginseng has been studied thoroughly except Siberian ginseng. It is necessary to purchase standardized ginseng that contains 15 percent ginsenosides. Ginseng that contains 15 percent ginsenosides indicates that manufactures have tested the product to ensure that there are sufficient quantities of the active chemicals. Most doctors recommend one to two grams a day. One word of caution here: Ginseng can cause a rise in blood pressure. Make sure you have your blood pressure tested regularly.

Avena Sativa: Avena sativa is a green oat straw that has been a staple of sex formulas for hundreds of years because of its ability to alleviate sexual problems and raise testosterone levels. Men taking 300 mg a day will have dramatic increases in the frequency of sexual activity.

Muira Puama: This is a herb that works both as an aphrodisiac and an erection booster. In one study, when 262 men took 1 to 1.5 g of muira puama daily for a period of two weeks, 51 percent reported better erections and 62 percent said it increased their libidos.[16]

L-Arninine: L-arginine is an essential amino acid and not an herb. It encourages the production of nitric oxide, a chemical that encourages penile blood flow. In a laboratory test, rats were fed this amino acid for eight weeks, which resulted in erectile responses. "The results is a lot like those seen with ginkgo-better blood flow to the genitals," says Steven Margolis, M.D., an alternative-medicine physician in Sterling Heights, Michigan. He suggest taking about 500 to 1000 mg daily.[17]

An ounce of Brazil nuts, peanuts, or almonds can give you sufficient amount of L-arginine. Also, soybeans, tofu and sunflower seeds are excellent sources of this dynamic amino acid.

St. John's Wort: St. John's Wort is a most popular herb since it acts as a natural antidepressant. So how can this herb help with your sex life? This herb will help with problems of depression, which may contribute to poor sexual functioning. Dr. Margolis says, "Obviously, if someone is depressed, he's going to have a decreased libido, and in that case St. John's Wort could be most helpful."[18] It is recommended to take 600 to 900 mg per day of 0.3 percent standardized extract.

Saw Palmetto: If you are a man over fifty years of age, it is most likely that you have an enlarged prostate gland. This bloated prostate gland could cause sexual problems by interfering with nerves and blood vessels that feed blood to the penis. "Prostate enlargement doesn't necessarily interfere with sexual function. But when it does, relieving the condition may help men attain an erection," says Dr. James Duke, Ph.D. author of *The Green Pharmacy* and a botanist who has spent nearly thirty years study in medicinal plants.[19] Saw palmetto has been known to greatly reduce the size of the swollen prostate with consistent usage over a period of time. It is recommend to take 320 mg a day if you have enlarged prostate. If you don't have a prostate condition, it actually could be detrimental to your sex life since it reduces the amount of testosterone.

Yohimbe: Yohimbe is the only herb of all the above that has advanced from being an alternative-medicine treatment to being a conventional prescription drug. Both the herb and drug work by dilating blood vessels, allowing more blood to flow to the penis. It is believed that it improves the blood flow to the lower region of the spinal cord, which facilitates the transmission of sexual stimuli.[20]

Too much yohimbe can be harmful and even fatal. Do not take this herb without consulting first with your primary care practitioner. Herbs can be absolutely wonderful or most harmful. As with anything, too much of a good thing can be harmful. Always make sure your doctor knows what you are taking and for the reason you are taking it!

Chapter 9

Sexual Problems
Women Encounter

God created women most uniquely with many myste-rious elements. Women are "beautifully and won-derfully made" and they are to be treated with care. Yet, as the little girl enters her teenage years, she will have years of menstruation ahead of her causing her to recon-sider how "wonderfully" she really feels especially if pre-menstrual syndrome is one of the problems. Then as the lady enters into the mid-forties, she will have to adjust to another life-style change called the menopause. This chap-ter is written to help a woman cope with these twin prob-lems by better nutrition and the adjustment needed dur-ing those times of her life.

There is a good nutritional approach to PMS (premen-strual syndrome) and menopause to aid women having these problems. Let us not forget that PMS is a real monthly hassle for many women. Men just don't have an under-standing of what women actually go through each month. One major difference between a man's body and a woman's is that the women's hormones are in a continu-ous state of flux. A man's sex hormones remain more stable until they are needed to engage in the sexual act. When a woman is about to menstruate, she experiences both physical and emotional changes in her body. It is estimated that over 90 percent of all women are said to have some form of premenstrual syndrome. Experts do not all agree to what extent women in America suffer from this natural monthly occurrence. Some claim as much as 58 percent experience PMS; others say that only 3 to 15 percent have this experience. We know that as many as 10 percent will seek medical advice for this problem. Some women become frightened by sharp fluctuations in mood and depression swings. Others are shocked by the weight gain that accompanies the monthly cycle.[1] These hormonal changes are not grasped by many women, which can cause unnecessary distress. The usual physical complaints are headache, bloating, fatigue, irritability and even insomnia.

Medical science believes that the causes of PMS are due largely to fluctuating hormonal irregularities during the monthly cycle. Often times symptoms will reoccur with regular predictions. As the cycle begins, the ovaries produce the female hormone called "estrogen." After ovulation, a second hormone, progesterone, appears on the scene. Progesterone is needful for pregnancy, but it affects the lining of the uterus (endometrium) causing it to become thicker, and swelling accompanies this condition. In addition, the general body tissues retain more sodium. Consequently, the sodium from salt draws more water and increases fluid build up. The space between the tissues swell and there is a weight gain. Other symptoms of PMS could be caused by swelling in the uterus, pelvis, abdomen, legs, liver, and brain.[2] Some women cope very well with PMS but to others it is a nightmare with much discomfort and emotional upheaval.

Confirmed medical research has shown that menstrual cramps are caused by a body chemical called prostaglandin.[3] The lining of the uterus contains this chemical but it is inhibited by the female hormone progesterone. This hormone is at peak levels about two weeks before the period begins. Its primary function is to help a nutrition-carrying blood supply reach the uterus on a monthly basis. The uterine wall blood buildup is God's way of preparation for pregnancy. When the brain receives information that the egg that has dropped is not fertilized, the progesterone level falls dramatically. Then the prostaglandin is released, so it can prompt the smooth muscles in the uterus to slowly return to normality. Thus, the blood lining is shed.

There are positive things you can do to help you through the monthly cycle. A change in diet and taking supplements will greatly reduce the symptoms of PMS.

Many plant extracts exhibit a tonic effect on the female hormonal system. It is believed that this tonic effect is the result from the action of phytoestrogens, as well as from the plant extract's ability to improve blood flow to the sexual organs.[4] The beauty of herbs is that they work to nourish and tone the female glandular and organ systems without having a drug effect. Because of this, many herbs become helpful in a broad range of female conditions.

Phytoestrogens are components of many medicinal herbs that have been used for hundreds of years. These conditions are now treated medically with the use of estrogen. Phytoestrogen containing herbs offer numerous advantages over the use of estrogens in the treatment of PMS and menopause. Both synthetic and natural estrogens may pose a significant health risks. It is believed that estrogens increase the risk of cancer, gallbladder disease and thromboembolic disease (strokes, heart attacks) while phytoestrogens have not been associated with any known side effects. It is known that phytoestrogens have the effect of limiting tumor growth in animals.

Phytoestrogens in herbs are capable of exerting estrogenic effects. The activity of phytoestrogens is only 2 percent as strong as estrogen.[5] Phytoestrogens exert a balancing action on the effects of estrogen. If estrogen levels are low, phytoestrogens add to the effects of estrogen. If the estrogen levels are high, phytoestrogens help reduce the estrogen effects.[6]

Due to the balancing actions of phytoestrogens on estrogen effects, both are recommended for PMS, menopause and menstrual abnormalities. Many of these herbs are known as "uterine tonics."

The four most important herbs used in the treatment of female disorders are: Dong quai (Angelica sinensis), licorice root (Glycyrrhiza glabra), chaste berry (Vitex agnus-castus) and black cohosh (Cimicifuga racemosa). These herbs have been used historically to lessen numerous symptoms of female complaints, including hot flashes.[7]

The chaste berry comes from the chaste tree, which is a native of the Mediterranean. Its berries have been used for centuries to relieve female complaints. Chaste berries were used to suppress the libido. Scientific studies have shown that the chaste berry has profound effects on pituitary function.[8] Its beneficial effects in menopause may be due to the alteration of pituitary function. The recommended dosage of the chaste berry is 30 to 40 milligrams of the seeds.

Another herb used in the fight of PMS and menopause is black cohosh. This herb was widely used by the American Indians and later by American colonists for the relief of menstrual cramps and menopause. Scientific studies have shown the benefits of black cohosh for the treatment of dysmenorrhea and menopause. Other clinical studies show that extracts of black cohosh relieve not only hot flashes but depression and vaginal atrophy.[9] This herb not only has vascular effects, but even reduces the hormone luteninizing (LH) levels. This has a positive effect on estrogen levels.

Unfortunately many post-menopausal women suffer from "vaginitis." Vaginal infections are six times more common than urinary tract infections.[10] Most women are able to distinguish between painful urination of a urinary tract infection and the external pain felt when urine passes over inflamed labial tissues.

In addition to causing physical discomfort and embarrassment, vaginitis maybe a symptom of something far more complicated. It could suggest a chronic inflammation of the cervix or a sexually transmitted disease. If infectious in nature, the agent may cause an ascending infection of the genital tract. This type of infection can lead to endometritis, salpingitis and pelvic inflammatory disease.[11] Chronic vaginal infections without symptoms have been implicated in recurrent urinary tract infections.

Some women are most reluctant to mention a vaginal infection to their doctors out of embarrassment. They feel this way since they believe that the doctor may think of them as having poor female hygiene or venereal disease. Nothing could be further from the truth.

It is so necessary to treat vaginitis since it could be a case of "Candida albicans," (also known as yeast infection), which has increased immensely since the early 1960's. This is due to the over prescribed antibiotics. There are now numerous predisposing factors for candidal vaginitis. The following may trigger a bout of vaginitis: allergies, antibiotics, diabetes mellitus, elevated vaginal pH, gastrointestinal candidiasis, oral contraceptives, nylon tights, pregnancy and steroids.[12]

The primary symptom of candidal vaginitis is vulval itching. In many cases, this itching is so severe that it prevents the woman from having intercourse. This is associated with the presence of a thick, curd-like or "cottage cheese" like discharge.[13] When this presence is found in the discharge, it is very strong evidence of a yeast infection.

The internal environment of the vagina is a reflection of the health of the entire female body.[14] Vaginal secretions are continuously released which affect the microbial flora. These secretions contain water, nutrients, electrolytes and proteins. The basic integrity of these secretions are affected by hormonal and dietary factors. A low meat or even a vegetarian diet is recommended for conditions of this nature. It is of the utmost importance to have a very healthy diet when dealing with vaginitis.

A diet high in Lysine containing foods and low in arginine containing foods will aid in reducing the reoccurrence of vaginitis. Some of the foods that are high in Lysine are yeast, chicken, tuna, turkey, halibut, beef, mung and lima beans, lentils, peanuts without skins, salmon, sardines, shrimp, chocolate and cheddar cheese. Some foods that are low in arginine are green beans, red beans, brown rice, cooked oatmeal, millet, whole milk, whole-wheat bread, and halibut.[15]

Vitamin A and Beta-carotene must be present in the diet to help build up the immune system. Thus, the frequencies of infections will be reduced. Beta-carotene is a source of non-toxic vitamin A precursors.[16] Beta-carotene has been shown to increase the number of active T cell numbers, which are necessary in fighting infection. Do not exceed the recommended dosage of these vitamins since there can be too much toxic waste produced from them. Pregnant women must be extremely cautious in taking vitamins A and beta-carotene. There could possibly be complications with pregnancies.

Vitamin B complex has proven to be beneficial in the treatment of vaginitis. The B complex vitamin combined with phytoestrogens has shown to be the most effective in the treatment of atrophiciginitis.

Vitamin C and bioflavonoids are essential nutrients needed for immune enhancement. A deficiency of Vitamin C reduces the bacteria-destroying activity of white cells. Vitamin C and bioflavonoids improve connective tissue integrity and reduce the spread of infection.[17]

Vitamin E is so essential for improved immune response. Experiments have shown that Vitamin E helps reduce some of the symptoms of menopause. Excessive intake of vitamin E does cause elevated blood pressure and one should never exceed 1,200 IU of vitamin E per day. Caution is needed when taking vitamin E.

Zinc is also necessary for good immune function. When zinc is low in the diet, the thymus gland does not work to its capacity. The thymus gland is essential in the making of killer T cells.

Garlic (Allium sativum) is antibacterial, antiviral and antifungal, and has even been shown to be effective against antibiotic-resistant organism.[18]

For The Proorgasmic Wife

Many married women have never experienced a total sexual response. However, that doesn't mean the sex should be less enjoyable for them than women who do have a total sexual response.

When a woman does not achieve a sexual response, feelings of frustration, self-doubt and inadequacy are stirred up. Consequently, the joy of climax seems less possible and feelings of failure become increasingly a reality. This woman does not comprehend that she can overcome this problem because she is plagued by memories of previous failures coupled with a lack of sexual knowledge. We should never forget that just because orgasm may not have been achieved, that does not mean that the woman is not full of love and warmth.

Often times sexual problems of this nature are rooted in the past, even before marriage. There is no need to seek the psychological cause of this unless it may be pertinent to your healing. Let us not forget that God is able to heal this problem. He created you and He loves you just as you are. First, seek the Lord about the love you have for your husband. Both of you will need to pray together about this issue seeking the wisdom of the Holy Spirit.

Recognize that neither your husband nor yourself is at fault. Start having a new understanding of your sexual relationship by realizing that you can achieve orgasm. Begin by loving your husband more affectionately and focusing on your marital relationship.

As you enter the physical aspect of your relationship, don't offer criticism of the other person's performance. This is a time of learning and a time of giving unselfishly. Your goal is to have a loving time in bed with your husband. The realization of your husband's loving pursuits can trigger a mental signal that will help build uninhibited sexual pleasure.[19]

If you desire to have an orgasm, recognize that several things must take place in your body before this happens. It is necessary to be sufficiently stimulated or nothing will take place. If your husband is not doing this, it is important to change the manner of your foreplay to ensure orgasm. At the same time, intense concentration is so important based upon your feelings and sensations. As you move with your feelings, desires and sensations, the likelihood of orgasm is more plausible.

It is so important to let your husband pursue orgasm with you. Let him work with you and both of you will find mutual satisfaction. Sex is from God and it is a good thing. As you are trying to enjoy your husband's advances, realize that you are not selfish by seeking personal fulfillment.

As you fulfill your desire, you too will be fulfilling your husband's needs and desires.

Simultaneous orgasm is wonderful, but it may not happen for some time. Do not let this stop you from enjoying sex with your husband. You have a lifetime to learn what pleases each other. Make each moment special and develop a love that lasts a lifetime. As you and your husband learn to mutually stimulate each other by touch and enjoyment of each other's body, orgasm and the joy of sex will abound.

If you are a woman who suffers from painful intercourse, please see your doctor. Painful intercourse is known as "dyspareunia." This is only a symptom of something else that your physician needs to investigate. Request a thorough physical examination, one that must include a pelvic and rectal examination.[20]

I hope that this information has provided you with a building block to create a healthier you. As you become a better lover, you will also become a woman who can lead her husband into deeper sexual fulfillment.

Chapter 10

Exercising to Enhance Your Sex Life

Any health professional will verify the importance of exercise in your life. Even taking a brisk walk at least five times a week for 20-30 minutes will benefit you physically as well as emotionally.

Whatever might have troubled you before, nothing can help you or cure you faster than a good brisk walk. It cannot cure everything, but walking causes the circulation to speed up the heart. It will take off the edge of various tensions, which will make good sex become more possible. Walking aids in relieving anxiety and everyday frustration. The rewards that walking offers equal those of such great sports as swimming and even snow skiing. Walking will help you lose weight and maintain your weight goal. Walking also helps in keeping bones strong and even improves your looks. Ultimately, when you feel better, your confidence in the bedroom improves. Walking allows a person to reflect on God and pray, and if done at night, it aids in relaxation and improves sleep.

Walking causes more oxygen to be taken into the bloodstream and allows arteries to become more elastic. Diet and exercise help prevent atherosclerosis and the tragic results of that disease.

Walking combined with a natural diet (vegetarian) is the best defense against the aging process. Remember, just because one may get older does not mean that sex is over. Walking also helps stimulate the intestines to function more quickly, which when accompanied by eating the right kinds of foods; it will help lower cholesterol and improve your love life.

Exercise will help reduce stress, which will increase sexual sensitivity. As one gets older, if exercise is not maintained the sex drive and enjoyment may become impaired.

If you have not been a walker, it is best that you start out slowly. It would even be advisable to consult your doctor before starting a walking program. Start with a short distance in which you will be comfortable. Take three to five days before you increase your distance. After a good week of walking, try to double your distance. If you increase your distance about 10 percent every three to four days, you will have doubled your distance in a very short time.[1] In the beginning, it's not important how fast you're walking. The speed will increase as your body becomes conditioned to walking, which will probably take about five weeks. If you are able to walk four or five miles in about five weeks time then you might try jogging.

Another benefit from walking is that the cost is minimal. All you need is a good pair of walking shoes and you're ready to go! Make sure your shoes fit well and are comfortable. Wear cotton or wool socks since they absorb perspiration.

Always be careful about your speed whether you are walking or jogging. Checking your heart rate is the best indication of your physical condition. If your pulse is 100 after walking or jogging for a minute then things appear to be just fine. If your pulse exceeds the 130 count, do less walking or jogging. When you're in shape your pulse should be around 100 beats per minute. It is important to monitor your heart rate so that you do not exceed your present level of activity until your heart is conditioned.[2]

While exercise may be a good thing for all of us, too much exercise can damage the joints, tear muscles and even damage the heart muscle. Various studies have shown that too much running, jogging or even weight lifting can diminish the sex drive.

Studies have shown that men or women who run up to forty miles a week may be burning off hormones as fast as they are consuming calories. With a loss of hormones is the possibility of a complete loss of the sex drive is feasible. This same thing can occur with weight lifters and those doing too much aerobic exercise. In order to compensate for this, a good nutritional program must be instituted followed by vitamin and mineral supplementation. Hormones must never be taken without the counsel of a good physician.

If you are exercising to lose weight, then it should be accompanied by a sensible diet and exercise plan tailored for you. As you begin to lose the weight, you will notice a greater intensity in your sex drive. Are you willing to take the time and energy needed to enhance it? This will take diligence on your part but it can be done and should be done just for the sake of your own body.

If you are under forty you can do strenuous exercise with your doctor's approval. If you are over fifty years of age, it is best not to do any type of strenuous exercise. Before starting a fitness program, consult your physician.

If you try walking, do it either in the morning before you have to be at your job or try walking after your evening meal. It will help with the digestion and give you time to reflect on your life.

Make a walking schedule so that you will make it a daily habit. During the winter, it is not always possible to walk outdoors but you sure can try walking in your local mall. Some malls across the country encourage people to walk by marking down a starting point and a finishing point. Ask your wife or husband or a good friend to walk with you and the both of you will benefit greatly.

Try parking your car a short distance from your place of work and walk the rest of the way. Instead of taking an elevator, try walking up the stairs for a change. This will strengthen your heart and increase your breathing capacity.

Always walk naturally and with a brisk pace while taking your walk. The average individual should be able to do about 120 steps after a good month of walking.

All aerobic teachers will tell you that your exercise program should include stretching and strengthening exercises. While doing your aerobic exercises you burn calories at a very fast rate. This is partially due to the metabolism speeding up by as much as 10 percent.

If you have a weight problem, be encouraged that aerobics burn more calories for heavy people than for thin individuals. At the same time, you will see your energy levels increased with better concentration and a sounder sleep.[3]

If weight loss is your goal, then aerobics are probably the best thing for you to do. Dancing, swimming, vigorous walking, cycling, roller skating, biking, running, power walking and cross-country skiing are excellent aerobic exercises. These burn fat at a faster rate because more energy is needed to do the exercise itself.

Many people benefit greatly from strength building exercises. You can even do strength building exercises while at the same time doing some of your aerobic workout. Most strength building programs are based on the use of freestanding weights. Barbells and dumbbells are used mainly for strengthening programs, but there are also specialized machines you can use at local fitness centers.

Another excellent exercise is jumping rope. Please know that jumping rope is not just for kids. It is also a cost efficient exercise. Agility, improved reflexes, toning your waist, hips and legs are the great results of being faithful to a jump rope exercise.[4]

Buy yourself a sturdy leather rope with wooden handles and find a good hard surface. Jump for three minutes, rest one minute, and then jump for another three minutes. This is more difficult than you can imagine. It is going to take some time before you can reach this level of exercise. If you count your warm-up exercises and cooldown time you're going to have a seven- to ten-minute fabulous aerobic workout.

Remember to keep your arms straightened at your sides, and swing the rope over your head using an easy wrist motion. Make sure your knees are slightly flexed and put a light spring in your toes. You can do all kinds of variations with the rope as you become skilled at this exercise.

Even with exercise and a well-balanced diet, there are those who find marital sex not too enjoyable. Women in particular may find intercourse painful or not pleasurable. A careful examination may show that this is correlated with flaccid, or "out of shape" musculature around the vaginal area.

There is an exercise that will help restore muscle tone in the pubococcygeus muscle.[5] It has been proven most successful to those women who faithfully practice this exercise. This exercise is known as "Kegels exercise." Firmly tense the muscles around your vagina and anus, as if you were stopping the flow of urine. Hold the contraction for as long as you can, working up to 6 to 10 seconds, allowing the muscles to relax completely between contractions.

Aim for ten to twenty repetitions two to three times each day. Strengthening these muscles will increase the joy of good sex.

When we take into consideration good exercise and a balanced diet, you are definitely going to have better sex. Not only will you feel better from exercise and a good diet, but you will look better too. In addition to this, it will help you to retain your youthfulness.

Chapter 11

Sex Is Always
Between Your Ears

Your mind is an incredible masterpiece. There isn't a computer on earth that can even begin to compare to the human mind.

Good sex begins right between our ears—in the mind—and ends with blissful pleasure between partners. Good sex must be giving and never one sided. God never intended that sex be an insult or something unclean to the spirit of man. Since some of us have been raised in Puritanical homes where sex was never mentioned, we have many misconceptions about sex. Consequently, as Christians, we were raised with "hang ups" about sex in general. Remember that God created sex and it is good. Christian sex in marriage should be expressed by being full of sensitivity in the context of real agape love. This will enable the couple to grow into a deep love relationship.

Consequently, we must really watch what comes into our minds because the mind is a battlefield. All day long things happen and at times we let down our mental guard. Many of our physical problems are directly related to what we are thinking or not thinking. Modern medicine recognizes that numerous physical diseases are truly psychosomatic in origin and that all illnesses have some basis as being psychosomatic.

The word *psychosomatic* comes from two Greek words *psyche* (mind) and *soma* (body). During the course of a day, all kinds of information is fed into the mind, and we have a choice to either accept what is being said or reject it. Nevertheless, some things affect us personally. Powerful emotions such as anger, hatred, bitterness or jealously have the potential to cause negative reactions in the body. Disease can result if we allow ourselves the luxury of entertaining such negative thoughts and emotions.

We must never underestimate the mind's influence in sexual malfunctions, sexual dissatisfaction, lovelessness, loneliness, deviation, glandular imbalances or any other aspect of human sexuality. We totally do not appreciate the mind's ability to cause sexual problems nor do we appreciate its ability to cure sexual difficulties. God, who is the solution to our problems, gives us the mental ability that will affect our sexual ability.

For successful sex in marriage, there must be a mutual mental agreement before there can be an agreement between bodies. When we don't take the time to spend time together, how can there be good sex? If a partner senses apathy or indifference, the initial reaction may be hurt, pain and feelings of rejection. Take time to know and enjoy your partner.

There are various influences in your life that will affect your mind to one degree or another. Things such as: genetic inheritance, childhood experience, education and home environment all play a contributing role to the good or poor functioning of the mind. It has been known for some time that nutrition can even influence the formation of the personality. To some degree we inherit personality traits from our primary caretakers (parents or guardians). All of these above-mentioned factors have influence on our minds.

Love is taught at an early age and is learned somewhat. As a child, if your parents showed you love and there was physical touching, you had a very blessed childhood. If your parents were good parents, but didn't show you the love necessary for critical self-esteem, you have had to learn how to love and overcome poor self-esteem. When there is no visible example of love toward the child, this particular child will have to overcome numerous difficulties in his or her life. Thank God that there is hope for this person because in Christ all things can be healed and sorted-out. Jesus Christ will teach you how to love.

When a child is denied the necessary love for emotional growth and development, we find this to be most detrimental to the conscious mind of that person. As a Christian counselor, I have dealt with individuals through the years who have experienced a loss of conscious. It is not easy for them to go through counseling but with the grace of God, they do learn how to change their behavior. They learn how to become loving people!

The scourge of the Christian church today is the number of partners filing for divorce who vowed before God and man that they would live as life-long partners. If parents would take into consideration the consequences of divorce in relationship to their children, they might think twice and seek healing of their marriage. Divorce upon children is caustic. It encourages such negative emotions as fear, abandonment, insecurity and loneliness. When these children become adults, often times they will be overly jealous, fearful and even tense about sexual intimacy. Isn't it time that parents realize the consequences of their actions upon their offspring?

It is time that the church of Jesus Christ starts teaching Christian Sex Education. When there is a godly approach toward sex education, many positive attitudes will enable the youngster to go through life with the right values. When sex education is taught in a public school, it is taught based on humanism—the philosophy of anything and everything is OK. This is the reason why we have such a high level of teenage pregnancies. Students being taught sex education in public schools are not taught the morality and necessity of staying pure until marriage.

It is not enough to inform children about sex. Morality of God's Word must be taught to our children. When sex education is taught in the public schools, there is an increase of sexually transmitted diseases. Consequently, today we have an epidemic of venereal herpes and AIDS.

Children must be taught that sex is more than just having a pleasurable feeling; it is sacred. Movies, television and the media present sex in such a light that the responsibility of such actions is never taken into consideration. The media never make any mention of the fact that man is more than just a body. Man is created in the image and likeness of God. Man is a spirit who lives in a human body. We are body, soul and spirit. These must be taken into account if our children are to be morally responsible people.

We need to feed our minds with good thoughts, music and even natural sounds. As human beings, we must have emotional satisfaction to become the people of God that He wants us to be. We need the right people to be around us who are not full of spite or bitterness. Above all else, we need to avoid negative people. At all times, we must deal honestly with those that are around us.

When we have a good relationship with Jesus Christ, our thought life is positive. It is important to watch carefully what we allow into our minds. Let the Lord have His way in your life and everything else will take on a whole new meaning.

Chapter 12

How Food and Mental Fatigue Affect Sexual Performance

The foods we eat give us energy, but many of our favorite foods can actually zap vital energy from our bodies. This is the result of being sensitive to a particular type of food or food groups.

There is a vast difference between food allergies and food sensitivities. Usually when the offending food is eaten, there is a rapid physical, allergic reaction to food, which causes the immune system to respond. Some physical symptoms might be: coughing, sneezing, rashes or hives, an intestinal disturbance and even more.[1] Whenever the food is eaten, there is a recognizable cause-and-effect relationship.

Food sensitivities are quite a different matter altogether. At one time "food sensitivities" were called "masked allergies" since the offending food reactions may not occur immediately.[2] Many people actually feel good after eating the offending food. This may appear contradictory, but examining this in the light of biochemistry of your body's stress response, it makes perfect sense. Once the stress response is triggered by hormones that are released into the blood stream causing a surge of energy and preparing the body for "fight or flight." When a food sensitivity reaction occurs, the body is overburdened in its attempts in trying to deal with the causative triggering food and the negative symptoms will appear. The reactions may occur as late as three to five days after eating offending foods.

Here are a few symptoms that occur to food sensitivities:

1. Chronic tiredness that never seems to go away;
2. Pressure in the head, headaches and even chest pains;
3. Excessive mucus secretion, sneezing and runny nose;
4. Abdominal gas pains, excessive flatulence, diarrhea and bowel disturbances;
5. Skin conditions such as: rash, skin irritations, eczema;
6. Poor sexual performance and the loss of sexual interest.[3]

It is important to understand that it is going to take a little time to identify the offending food. If you have an idea that a certain food does not agree with you, try taking it out of your diet for five or six days. This will enable you to see if there is positive change. If your symptoms disappear, try adding that food back to your diet just to observe what happens.

If you have a craving for different foods, make a list of them. Usually the most common foods that contribute to food sensitivities are: wheat, corn, tomatoes, cane sugar, chocolate, fish, chicken, cow's milk, yeast, cheese, bacon, artificial food additives and food colorings.

Modern nutritional research has shown us that a diet of meat, potatoes, cream, cheese, butter and white bread is terribly wrong. A diet high in fat, sugar and protein and low in complex carbohydrates and fiber can lead to such diseases as cancer, high blood pressure, heart disease, clogged arteries, diabetes, osteoporosis and arthritis. Such a diet robs you of much needed energy and leaves you feeling sluggish. The body has to work overtime to get the poisons out of it. Consequently, there is little energy left to do anything else. In order to have good sex you must start with a good diet.

Soft drinks are loaded with white sugar, which puts a severe strain on the immune system. Soft drinks will contribute to chronic tiredness, which hinders anyone from having good sex. Even with the use of diet soft drinks, these too will cause unusual tiredness because they are filled with artificial colorings, flavorings and sweeteners. Diet soft drinks are also loaded with sodium, which leads to water retention giving you a bloated feeling.

Caffeine

Caffeine will cause the immune system to be overstimulated. Let's take a good look at coffee. After a cup of coffee you feel great until you crash after overstimulation. So then you have another cup of coffee, and by the end of the day, you've had four to six cups of coffee! After a period of years, overstimulation of the immune system will cause it to break down. This abuse of the fight-or-flight stimulation of the immune system will only leave you further tired, sluggish and no good for sex. Stop drinking coffee! If you can't stop drinking it, then gradually reduce the number of cups per day to one or two. This will help increase mental alertness. I used coffee as an example, but there are other "caffeine culprits": chocolate, tea and caffeinated soft drinks. Caffeine not only leads to overstimulation, but it also dehydrates your body of its necessary fluids.

You may be experiencing tiredness and loss of body fluids due to your work environment or even in your home. The central heat in your home or workplace depletes your body of much needed moisture. Perhaps you work in an office and hardly have a chance to get outside during the day. A dehydrated body could be one of the many reasons you're tired and have lost interest in personal intimacy with your partner. Try replacing the fluids in your body by bringing a bottle of water to work. (It's best to drink pure distilled water if possible.) Stay away from drinking caffeinated beverages or alcohol that will drain the body of necessary fluids since they act as diuretics. If your don't like pure water, try drinking carbonated water. This kind of water does absorb into the body very rapidly but also causes belching.

Mental Aerobics

Most Americans lead a fast-paced lifestyle that can zap the energy right out of the body.

If you're an office worker or you spend hours in your car, these types of activities cause mental and muscle fatigue. Ridding yourself of fatigue isn't easy, but instead requires daily exercise to be free of the effects of this kind of lifestyle. Muscle tension can result from having a sedentary job. The muscles of the upper back, neck shoulders, face and forehead are tensed more than what you may be aware, and the result is a lessening of needed oxygen that needs to flow through the muscle and even the brain.[4] Consequently, there is less blood and oxygen for tensed muscles, which means there is less nourishment for the involved muscles. Lactic acid builds up with waste products resulting in that "old tired feeling."

Perhaps you come home from work stressed out and try to have sex just before going to bed but the results may not be what you anticipated. This is totally understandable since performance is inhibited by accelerated stress. The only way to avoid this situation is to exercise four or five times a week. Exercise will alleviate the accumulated stress and assist you in better sexual performance.

When the brain doesn't get enough oxygen for peak performance, the result is mental fatigue. Mental fatigue leaves one unable to think clearly, results in temporary memory loss and feeling mentally "exhausted." If we are to have peak sexual performance in our marriages, we need to learn how to get more oxygen out of our exercises sessions, which will cause greater amounts of oxygen to get to the brain. Remember all good sex begins in the brain. You cannot have good sex if the brain is constantly fatigued.

Most of us don't know that we are creatures of body rhythms and cycles. I first learned this in 1976 when Rita and I traveled to the United Kingdom. It was an especially long journey since we had to travel to Canada from Texas. After leaving Toronto, Canada, we flew to London's Heathrow Airport. We had crossed at least six time zones. I was to learn that "jet lag" is very real and it was going to take us a good week to overcome our strange new feelings. We were sleeping when we should have been awake; we were awake when we should have been sleeping. We are tied up with the twenty-four-hour cycle called the "circadian cycle" based upon earth's twenty-four-hour cycle or rotation.[5] If this cycle is changed somehow by taking a long journey, the body will respond accordingly. Certain times of the day we have more energy than at other times. Even our heart rate and blood pressure is affected if we don't follow our natural rhythm patterns. Consequently, if you are a night worker, you are going to experience much fluctuation in your bodily rhythms. This can only lead to additional tiredness and poor sexual performance.

Within our twenty-four-hour cycle personal differences will affect all of us. Some of us perform better during the day while others will perform better at night. Maybe you're at a job feeling absolutely drained, but you might experience an energy burst once you're home. Time change and diet are things that ultimately affect how we relate to others, especially our mate.

Women especially understand what it means to have a monthly cycle. They comprehend the meaning of "fluctuation": moods, energy levels and food cravings are definitely affected during the menstrual cycle. The female cycle can have a tremendous influence on a woman's performance at work and at home.

Very few people realize that the human body is affected by the cycles of the four seasons. Many people talk about "spring fever" but what they don't understand is that the body prepares itself to lower its temperature in response to the warmth of the weather. The blood begins to thin and people tend to feel more tired than usual. At the same time, when the weather is much hotter in the summer, most people have greater amounts of energy. People are also stay out in the sunlight more, which also gives the body energy. It is also a known fact that people eat lighter foods in the summer than during the seasons of cold weather. All this results in better sexual performance during the summer months.

It has been known for over two hundred years that the flow of blood in the human body is affected by the phases of the moon. Some surgeons will not operate during a full moon because they know that the person is more likely to develop a bleeding condition.[6] We need to become more aware of the times of the day when we experience greater levels of energy. If we are cognizant of our energy levels, sex will be more pleasurable.

It is so important to feed the brain the correct foods that will produce greater brain performance. We must spend time in knowing what is best for our brains since the brain must have good nutritious foods to produce a constant nerve supply. If we don't have the right nerve supply, nothing else really matters. Hair has a problem in growing if the nerve supply to the scalp is deficient. Breathing becomes more difficult if the nerve supply in inadequate. The digestion of food and even the necessary amounts of hydrochloric acid will be insufficient unless the nerve supply is correct.[7] The body's sexual system works in conjunction with the nerve supply. The foods that feed the brain and those that feed the sexual system are virtually the same. The choice of foods must be selected from natural, pure and whole foods.

Sexual balance is so necessary. Our sexual glands must be taken care of just like any other gland found in the body. How are the sex glands fed properly? First, there has to be good thinking on the part of the individual. If the mind is filled with filth, it will be detrimental to good sex. Watch with what kinds of friends you associate. We all need to have good friends around us at times so that we receive positive, life-building words that encourage and edify us.

For good brain function and good sexual function, the role of vitamin E cannot be over stressed. Many of us have gone through life with a drug approach for health and healing. Countless surgeries have been performed on women which really may not have been necessary. There is such a high percentage of hysterectomies performed on women that could have been avoided if proper nutrition would have been given through the years. Many of these operations might have been avoided if Vitamin E and other related vitamins and minerals had been supplied. Vitamin E aids in keeping the sexual system in balance.

It should be understood from the very start that you cannot do just what you want with your sexual system. There has to be moderation and balance. Sexual energy can be channeled into your spiritual life and used for the mental and spiritual activity you enjoy in life.[8] Vitamin E works in conjunction with the nervous system for good functioning.

Nerve force and proper nutrients for the nervous system must be stressed. Nerve force can easily be built up with a growing relationship with Jesus Christ. Our Lord brings inner peace and happiness to the one who will take the time to be in His presence. The joy of the Lord is electrical and contagious! Happiness comes from His presence bringing harmony to the whole body. The wonderful harmony can be depleted by throwing it away if there is sexual excess. Remember the powerful emotions of hate, anger, fear and jealousy can disturb the chemical balance. If this should happen good sex becomes more difficult with your mate. There must come a time in our lives where we choose to live above such negativity. The choice will help the body and all of its glands to recuperate and even last longer.

Another factor both for good brain function and good sexual function is the role that zinc plays in the diet. For about the last twenty years there has been considerable interest in the role of the trace mineral zinc It is present in human tissues but most importantly it is found in the sexual organs and the thyroid. A newborn infant will have several times the amount of zinc in their liver as compared to an adult.

Zinc is so essential for the production of the male reproductive fluid. Zinc is made in the pancreas, the large gland located behind the lower part of the stomach, where it aids in the storage of glycogen. Glycogen is an energy producing substance. Zinc combines with phosphorus to assist in respiration. Zinc also causes vitamins to be broken down more rapidly. This mineral helps with the intake of oxygen and expulsion of carbon dioxide as toxic wastes. Zinc aids in the functioning of insulin. But when there is a shortage of insulin, it can lead to diabetes.[9] When there is sufficient amounts of zinc in the diet, food absorption occurs more readily through the intestinal wall. Zinc is part of a stomach enzyme. This wonderful vitamin plays a powerful role in the production of male hormones. Since the mineral is intimately connected with carbohydrate utilization, a deficiency of zinc may cause chronic fatigue. Remember that zinc produces energy.

One other important mineral needed for good sexual performance is manganese. Manganese works with the B-complex vitamins to overcome laziness, sterility and aids in sexual performance in men and women. It also combines with phosphatase, an enzyme, to assist in bone building. The mineral may be found in liver. Manganese is needed for good enzymatic function so foods may be digested and vital nutrients extracted for overall body utilization.[10] Manganese helps build resistance to various diseases and helps make strong nerves. In the pregnant mother this wonderful mineral helps promote milk formation.

Manganese can be found in green leaves, peas, beets and egg yolks. It may be found in unmilled grains. Another good source of manganese is sunflower seeds.

What governs our daily thought life is so essential for good love and good sex. As the apostle Paul mentions in Philippians 4:8: "Finally, brethren, whatever things are true, whatever things are noble, whatever things are just, whatever things are pure, whatever things are lovely, whatever things are of good report, if there is any virtue and if there is anything praiseworthy-meditate on these things."

We can know all about vitamins, minerals and herbs but these are only a part of a lifestyle. God has called us to a life with goodness. Our lives must be filled with the Holy Spirit and it is He that brings harmony to our mind (soul) and body. When our spirits are in harmony with our minds (souls) our bodily functions and appetites will bring the greatest of physical joys-and good sex.

Chapter 13

They Shall Be One Flesh

When a young couple stands before the minister and the altar of God, and accepts and receive vows they enter God's perfect covenant. Soon they will become "one flesh," experiencing new joys and pleasures of intimacy on their honeymoon. This is God's ideal.

As this takes place, the young couple begins a learning process before God where they will teach each other the way to achieve maximum enjoyment and pleasure. There comes a time of great understanding between the both of them which should expand over their entire lifetime. They may begin with some powerful information about sex but soon learn there is much more to sexual intimacy than they realized.

Some young couples enter marriage with the idea that they know all about sex only to find themselves totally frustrated because their knowledge was either insufficient or not appropriate. Young couples need to seek premarital Christian counseling in the area of sex and sexual relationships since what they know may not lead to sexual fulfillment. God has designed marriage to keep all of us from loneliness and He designed sex in marriage for pleasure and gratification. In marriage the couple is to become one in spirit, soul and body.

So many couples can relate in spirit and soul but cannot adequately relate in their bodies. Many Christian marriages are incomplete since they cannot relate to each other in a sexual manner. If they do so, it is not as pleasing as it might be.

Secular presentation of sexual intimacy through media presents the world's interpretation, which is often crude and unbecoming in its enfoldment. Christians need to have a Christian interpretation of what sex is all about, especially sexual intimacy.

When having sex as a couple, it is necessary to have total privacy. If there are children at home, they should be taught to respect the privacy of their parent's bedroom while the door is shut. If necessary, have a lock on the door that will prevent intrusion. In addition, children should not be allowed to sleep with their parents. Of course, if there is an infant, it is perfectly permissible to have the baby in the bedroom for the first four months.

The atmosphere in the bedroom should be romantic and relaxing. But the most important thing about sexual intercourse is that both people are enjoying each other's bodies. And keep the TV out of the bedroom!

Sexual arousal is a set of bodily responses making both partners ready for sexual intercourse. There is a wide range or variety of stimuli that may bring this about.[1] This time of sexual stimulation is called foreplay, which should be a most delightful time for both partners. The couple should be tender to each other by demonstrating their love for one another. The wife enjoys being caressed and wooed by her husband. At the same time the husband should appreciate his wife's advances toward him and accept them graciously. The couple should not rush this time of fore-play, but enjoy the moment.

Arousal is the result of reflex nerve responses to stimulation of parts of the skin rich in nerve ending.[2] The most sensitive areas of the body are called the erogenous zones. These include the genitals, abdomen, buttocks and the thighs. A woman's most responsive area of her body is the clitoris, while the man's is the lower side of the head of the penis. Other sensitive parts of the body are the lips, tongue, eyes, nose, nipples and breasts, which all play an important role in sexual arousal. Gentle touching, stroking, kissing or even blowing on one or more parts of the erogenous zones will cause definite arousal of the penis and the clitoris.

Intercourse should always draw the couple together and never apart. All kinds of emotions of love and goodness are spilled over as the couple experiences the bliss of orgasm. It should be noted that often times most women view intercourse quite differently than men. Women see intercourse and their sexual relationship with their husbands as a total package of the entire relationship. Men think of their sexual relationships with their wives as being something separate from the rest of their relationship. The glorious part about sex is both partners accepting responsibility in giving and receiving, then dynamic love is expressed for each other. It is impossible to delete daily behavior from your sexual union. Daily behavior can either make or break the beauty of intercourse. A wife who has been abused in any way by her husband during the day will not find beauty in the act of intercourse with him in the evening. The husband who has been controlled and nagged at by his wife at the breakfast or dinner will not enjoy the richness of intercourse.

Since the nerve endings vary from individual to individual, some couples soon find parts of the body more sensitive than others do. Even manipulation of the non-erogenous parts of the body can cause arousal since the partner has learned to associate this kind of touching with intercourse.

Kissing, embracing, petting and even fondling are part of a glorious foreplay. As each partner touches the other partner's body in a caressing manner, perfect arousal begins and ends in joyous intercourse. All parts of the body should be considered as sacred when touching and caressing takes place. Tell each other what feels the best and do not be embarrassed about this holy act of sex fulfillment. Solomon said, "Thou art all fair, my love, there is no spot in thee" (Song of Solomon 4:7). Solomon's wife responded, "He is altogether lovely. This is my beloved, and this is my friend" (5:16).

Take time to enjoy each other. Once sexual stimulation is nearing its peak, it is important for each other to carry through with the process so fulfillment will ensure. Let your body move gently in touching your partner's, which will heighten sexual excitement.

Each partner must learn to control his or her timing of sexual response. The wife especially should trust her husband and relate to him how she feels, this way; both may experience climax at the same time. This takes practice, but marriage allows for such practice. As the wife relates her feelings during intercourse, the husband will be enabled to time more adequately his orgasm.

Remember, during and after sexual intercourse there are marked changes in both male and female organs. These changes or alterations of the organs take place in varying stages of the corresponding four phases of intercourse: excitement, plateau level, orgasm and resolution.[3] The main functions of these changes are enabling the penis to penetrate the vagina; making the vagina receptive to the penis; and releasing sperm to fertilize an ovum. Upon completion of intercourse called "resolution," the sex organs return to normal size over a period of time.[4]

Often times it is most beneficial for women to use a lubricant for enhanced sexual stimulation, especially if the wife is unable to produce enough natural lubricant. The clitoris that has been well lubricated is more likely to be more responsive to the husband's penis. Attempting intercourse while the vagina is dry is very difficult for both partners especially for the husband since the tightness of the vagina may cause him to lose his erection.

Often times in counseling I am asked what is the best position for intercourse. There are many and numerous positions that couples might use but not all are comfortable for the female partner.

Briefly, the most common position is the "missionary" or "matrimonial" position. This is the position where the husband is on top of his wife in a face-to-face position. This was the most common position used unto the later part of the 1900's.

The missionary position is most adaptable than many other positions. This type of intercourse maybe shallow or deep and even prolonged. Couples find that this position tends to assist in mutual orgasm.[5] With the missionary position, there are variations that may be used to bring further enjoyment.

The opposite of the missionary position is face-to-face with the wife on top of her husband. This position is especially good for the men who may have experienced back injuries and find it difficult in any other position. This allows the wife for free control and length of the sexual union and both individuals may intensify intercourse if they so desire during this position. The wife can even start to kneel and shift to lying or other positions without losing control or contact.[6]

Another position used by partners today is the side-by-side position. There are many advantages of side-by-side intercourse including that neither partner bears the other's weight and both partners are totally free to embrace each other unencumbered. Couples find these positions unsatisfactory since they offer little scope for stimulation.[7]

Some couples practice rear-entry positions. It's mostly men who find this position most enjoyable while women find it rather impersonal. The disadvantage to this position is that neither partner may see each other's face. For the man rear entry offers satisfying deep penetration. Rear entry does put a lot of pleasing pressure on the clitoris.[8] Rear entry may be performed by kneeling, sitting and even standing. Some people find rear entry most enjoyable since they have medical conditions that may rule out other methods of intercourse. Rear entry positions are most beneficial when the wife is pregnant.

The next stage is the climax, where orgasm is reached. The word *orgasm* comes from the Greek word *orge*, which means "excitement." In the woman's body it is has been described as a momentary feeling of suspension followed by a rush of warmth starting in the perineal area and flowing through the entire body.[9] The lower third of the vagina begins to contract causing numerous other contractions—from three to ten—within a period. The intensity of this maybe increased by voluntarily strengthening her P.C. muscle contractions while she allows her own pelvic movements to correspond to her husband's movements. As her mental concentration is focused on orgasm, her total satisfaction is reached by coming to a complete satisfying climax. This is often a most intensified emotional experience of joy.[10]

The husband's orgasm consists of involuntary muscle tension and contractions. There are great sensations in the penis, prostate and seminal vesicles. In both sexes, the experience of orgasm is centered in the pelvic area of the body. The women experience sensations in the clitoris, vagina and uterus. Intense sensations are felt as a flood throughout the body. The major physical difference between the male and female orgasm is that men emit and ejaculate sperm and women do not.

After sexual intercourse, the fires of passion begin to calm down. As this takes place there seems to be a lovely, quiet glow of satisfaction. This is the time that each partner needs to show tenderness and love. Lying close together and gently patting or stroking the other brings greater closeness. Perhaps as much as fifteen minutes is needed for both partners to come back to a place of normalcy. The younger men may find that more time maybe needed for their erection to disappear.[11]

Each partner should become an expert on pleasing his or her mate. King Solomon said, "I am my beloved's, and his desire is toward me" (Song of Solomon 7:10).

Epilogue

Shaping Your Love Life

In order to be a good lover, many times we need to awaken our inner person both to give and receive love. We need to take a good look at self so that we might become the lover we need to be for our spouse. This is not a selfish goal but a realistic one. Perhaps there are areas of your inner development that need to be investigated so that further growth may take place. Only Christ can change you. Truly we need to know ourselves and love ourselves.

Your whole life in Christ now is the result of your thinking. By recognizing why you are the way you are, you will unlock the door that has kept back the real you from becoming the person you want to be in Christ. So many Christians concentrate on the negative aspects of their beings that they seldom think of what they have received in Christ. Many of us come into the Christian experience with a negative view of ourselves because we've been conditioned since we were children to think in such a manner. So many experience the love of God but do not know how to share personal love with their partner. False values, beliefs and the inability of sharing love have kept us back from realizing who we are in Christ and how truly capable we are in Him.

By virtue of the New Birth we have the power of God's Holy Spirit to change our lives totally for the good. We have the power through God's Word to begin to live in the "now" of things and enjoy who we truly are. It is in the process that we can experience love and give love to our partners without any reservation.

"For God so loved the world that He gave His only begotten Son, that whosoever believeth in Him should not perish, but have everlasting life" (John 3:16).

Do you realize that there is eternal life flowing in your veins? Are you aware of the fact that the same mighty Holy Spirit who worked in the resurrection of the Lord Jesus Christ is in your spirit man? All the power that was used in the resurrection of our Lord Jesus is in *you* this very day if you are born again. You can change in becoming a more sensitive loving and giving person. God's Spirit has the power to change you if you so desire.[1]

Because of the power of the New Birth and by the grace of the Lord, you are able to change every aspect of your being. You can do this as the Holy Spirit gives you insights into your personality, which need a conscious effort on your part to change. The Great Problem Solver abides within you. Every problem that might come across your path has a proper solution that the Holy Spirit will show you. This includes all problems as well as the inability in sharing yourself with your mate. He can help you in these matters.[2]

The Word of God teaches us that "The Kingdom of God abides within you" (Luke 17:21). It is not in some distant continent but it is within you. Because of this wonderful truth there are self-healing powers available to those who seek the Holy Spirit as He abides in them. Health, happiness, abundance and peace of mind are within each believer who seeks to be free from the shackles of previous conditioning.

Unless you begin to see your self-worth as a person, you cannot even begin to see yourself in Christ as you should. Only to the degree that you accept your self-worth in Christ Jesus as a person will you be able to free yourself from self-imposed chains of slavery. As this takes place your ability to give and receive love will be increased, and as a result, you certainly will enjoy life a lot more.

If you cannot surrender your guilt feelings and feelings of inadequacy to Christ, you will be one of those who continues the endless struggle to attain self-confidence and true sexual fulfillment. To enjoy the freedom of the Lord and be a warm, compassionate, loving person, you must begin by examining your heart in the light of God's Word. To follow Luke's advice "Love thy neighbour as thyself" without having an understanding of who you are, is to underestimate yourself and what you can become in Christ. It also has the effect of underestimating the value of your neighbor.

Some may consider what is being said here is totally unchristian and completely selfish. A closer examination of what is being said here will only shed further light on Luke's admonition: "Love thy neighbour as thyself" (Luke 10:27). It is imperative to see that first you need to identify your personal needs and then those of your neighbor. Realize that it is not your business to please others first by yourself. This may sound very unpious, but a closer look will show you how important it is. It is only as you have done the very best by God's grace to make the most of yourself that you can be the greatest value to your spouse, family, friends and church.

To be a good lover, you have to love yourself in a healthy and wholesome manner. The most important fact to consider is that Jesus Christ by His grace can change you. From being afraid to love or not knowing how to love, His grace will assist you in understanding who you are and what you are in Him. As you yield yourself to Jesus Christ, inner healing will come. It is in this process of giving that you can take control of your life through Jesus Christ. (See John 12:24.) As we please Him, giving our inner person to Christ, the blockages and pains of un-filled yesterdays are healed and you become less emotion-ally restrained. This will be reflected in a new tenderness and love for your marital partner.

Many adults have difficulty in loving another and even with the expression of physical love in their sex life. Usu-ally this can be traced back to an early childhood trau-matic event. How a child learns the facts of life will greatly influence his love and ability to relate to the opposite sex as an adult.

When children are subjected to any type of child abuse, this can remain with them the rest of their lives if Christ is not allowed to heal those wounds. Nor are we able to ignore the damage that divorce has on a child. If a child witnesses physical or verbal abuse the effects of these are very damaging. Often these adults are ill advised to seek spiritual counseling from one trained in these problems. All of the negative aspects that may have occurred during the early formative years will manifest itself in the adult in one way or another.

Children are most impressionable and their little minds are like computers recording everything in detail to be replayed someday later on. We must take time in show-ing our love for our children and repeatedly tell them how much we love them. Children learn how to love with as-surance of parental love and children grow into well-rounded adults who know how to enjoy their lives.

Many adults do not know how to love. Adults that lack skills in the realm of love will need to learn to love. They will need to consciously seek counsel in developing their love skills. Many will have to learn to listen to the Holy Spirit within them as He moves them along a road of true education.

There is a very good remark that is so very poignant, "Que sera, sera (Whatever will be, will be)." In other words, regardless of past mistakes or personal tragedies, these must not be allowed to dominate our present moment. Through Jesus Christ life can start all over again. This is a new day, old habits can be broken, and new ways of living in a warm, loving manner can be learned. Past tragedies can be healed by the power of the Holy Spirit. There is a new dawn for those who choose to awaken to it.

There is no better way to learn to love than in helping others. As we see the needs of others, we tend to love ourselves more readily. In Christ we are called to be servants. What does a servant do? He helps his master at whatever task is at hand. Our Master Jesus Christ has called us to love our neighbor. We can do this by assisting people in whatever capacity we are able.

Loving service lifts us out of our depression. The end product of which is a positive self-esteem. As this takes place, we are enabled to enter the real joy of Jesus Christ. This has been our Lord's goal all the time—the perfect harmony of spirit, soul and body. This is the best and only way to live.

Notes

Chapter One

To Attract or Not to Attract

1. Ed Wheat, M.D. and Gaye Wheat, *Intended For Pleasure*, (Old Tappan, NJ: Fleming H. Revell Company, 1981), 20.

2. Bernard Jensen, Dr., *Love, Sex & Nutrition*, (Garden City Park, NY: Avery Publishing Group Inc., 1988), 30.

Chapter Three

Our Faulty Diets

1. *Mosby's Medical Dictionary*, 4th ed. (1994), s.v. "Hypothalamus."

2. Bernard Jensen, Ph.D., *Love, Sex & Nutrition*, (Garden City Park, NY: Avery Publishing Group, Inc., 1988), 11.

3. James E. Marti, *Alternative Health Medicine Encyclopedia*, (Detroit, MI: Visible Ink Press), 126.

4. Ibid., 126.

5. Ibid., 126.

6. Ibid., 126.

7. Ibid., 126.

Chapter Four

Minerals Make Things Work Better

1. Carlson Wade, *Magic Minerals*, (West Nyack, NY: Parker Publishing Company, Inc., 1968), 3.

2. Ibid.

3. Ibid.

4. Ibid., 5.

5. Ibid., 4.

6. Ibid., 3.

7. Ibid., 4

8. Ibid., 4.

9. Bernard Jensen, Dr., *Love, Sex & Nutrition,* (Garden City Park, NY: Avery Publishing Group Inc., 1988), 136.

10. Carlson Wade, *Magic Minerals,* 18.

11. Bernard Jensen, Dr., *Love, Sex & Nutrition,* 137.

12. Carlson Wade, *Magic Minerals,* 18.

13. Ibid., 19.

14. Ibid., 19.

15. Bernard Jensen, Dr., *Love, Sex & Nutrition,* 143.

16. Ibid., 141.

17. Ibid., 141.

18. Carlson Wade, *Magic Minerals,* 22.

19. Ibid., 23.

20. Don Colbert, M.D., *Walking in Divine Health,* (Lake Mary, FL: Creation House, 1999), 175.

21. Carlson Wade, *Magic Minerals,* 26.

22. Ibid., 27.

23. Ibid., 26

24. Ibid., 24.

25. Ibid., 25.

26. Bernard Jensen, Dr., *Love Sex and Nutrition,* 145.

27. Ibid., 146.

Chapter Five

God-given Vitamins for a Joyous Sex Life

1. Dr. Bernard Jensen, *Love Sex & Nutrition,* (Garden City Park, NY: Avery Publishing Group, 1988) 152.

2. James F. Balch, M.D. and Phyllis A. Balch, C.N.C., *A-Z Guide to Supplements,* (Garden City Park, NY: Avery Publishing Group, 1998), 34.

3. Ibid., 35.

4. Dr. Bernard Jensen, *Love, Sex & Nutrition,* 154.

5. James F. Balch, M.D. and Phyllis A. Balch, C.N.C., *A-Z Guide To Supplements,* 36.

6. Ibid., 38.

7. Ibid., 38.

8. Dr. Bernard Jensen, *Love, Sex & Nutrition,* 155.

9. James F. Balch, M.D. and Phyllis A. Balch, C.N.C., *A-Z Guide To Supplements,* 39.

10. Dr. Bernard Jensen, *Love, Sex & Nutrition,* 157.

11. James F. Balch, M.D. and Phyllis A. Balch, C.N.C., *A-Z Guide To Supplements,* 46.

12. Ibid., 47.

13. Ibid., 47.

14. Ibid., 48.

15. Dr. Bernard Jensen, *Love, Sex & Nutrition,* 159.

Chapter Six

Glorious Nutrients for a Better Sex Life

1. George Halpern, MD, Ph.D., *Ginkgo, A Practical Guide,* (Garden City Park, NY: Avery Publishing Group, 1998), 120.

2. Ibid., 121.

3. Ibid., 121.

4. Ibid., 121.

5. Charles B. Clayman, M.D., "Impotence," *Encyclopedia of Medicine,* (NY: Random House, 1989) 578.

6. Ibid., 578.

7. George Halpern, MD, Ph.D., *Ginkgo-A Practical Guide,* 123.

8. Ibid., 123.

9. Bernard Jensen, Dr., *Love, Sex & Nutrition,* (Garden City Park, NY: Avery Publishing Group Inc., 1988), 192.

10. Ibid., 192.

11. Ibid., 192.

12. Ibid., 194.

13. Peggy Canning, M.S., *Exotic Supplements,* (Vista, CA: Margaret H. Canning, 1996), 18.

14. Bernard Jensen, Dr., *Love, Sex & Nutrition,* 193.

Chapter Seven

Your Glands and Good Sex

1. Charles B. Clayman, M.D., *The American Medical Association Encyclopedia of Medicine,* s.v. "Endocrine System" (NY: Random House Inc., 1989).

2. Bernard Jensen, Dr., *Love, Sex & Nutrition,* (Garden City Park, NY: Avery Publishing Group Inc., 1988), 60.

3. Ibid., 60.

4. Ibid., 61.

5. Charles B. Clayman, *The American Medical Association Encyclopedia Of Medicine,* s.v. "Pituitary Gland."

6. Bernard Jensen, *Love, Sex & Nutrition,* 61.

7. Charles B. Clayman, *The American Medical Association Encyclopedia Of Medicine,* s.v. "Thyroid Gland."

8. Bernard Jensen, *Love, Sex & Nutrition,* 61.

9. Charles B. Clayman, *The American Medical Association Encyclopedia Of Medicine,* s.v. "Pineal Gland."

10. Bernard Jensen, *Love, Sex & Nutrition,* 61.

11. Ibid., 61.

12. Ibid., 61.

13. Charles B. Clayman, *The American Medical Association Encyclopedia Of Medicine,* s.v. "Prostate Gland."

14. Ibid., "Pancreas."

15. Bernard Jensen, *Love, Sex & Nutrition,* 61.

16. Charles B. Clayman, *The American Medical Association Encyclopedia Of Medicine,* s.v. "Ovary."

17. Ibid., "Testis".

18. Ibid., "Hypothalamus".

19. *Mosby's Medical Dictionary,* s.v. "Prostaglandins," (St. Louis, MO: Mosby - Year Book, Inc., 4th ed., 1994).

20. Charles B. Clayman, *The American Medical Association Encyclopedia Of Medicine,* s.v. "Puberty."

21. Berry Sears, Ph.D., *The Anti-Aging Zone,* (Regan Books, HarperCollins Publishers, New York, 1999), 252.

22. Ibid., 252.

23. Ibid., 252.

24. C. Norman Shealy, M.D., Ph.D., *DHEA The Youth And Health Hormone,* (New Canaan, CT: Keats Publishing,

Inc., 1996), 36.

25. Ibid., 36.

26. Ibid., 36.

27. Ibid., 37.

28. Ibid., 38.

29. Ibid., 42.

30. Ibid., 43.

31. Peggy Canning, M.A., *Exotic Supplements,* (Vista, CA: Margaret H. Canning, 1995), 28.

32. Ibid., 28.

33. Ibid., 28.

Chapter Eight

Male Sexual Problems and the Prostate

1. Carlson Wade, *Nutritional Healers,* (West Nyack, NY: Parker Publishing Company, Inc., 1987), 181.

2. Ibid., 182.

3. Ibid., 182.

4. *Sex: A User's Manual,* (New York, NY: Berkley Publishing Company, 1982), 242.

5. Ibid., 244.

6. Ibid., 245.

7. *The Harper Collins Illustrated Medical Dictionary,* 1993 ed. s.v. "Prostatitis."

8. *Encyclopedia of Medicine,* 1989 ed., s.v. "Prostatitis."

9. Carlson Wade, *Nutritional Healers,* 185.

10. Ibid. 186.

11. Ibid., 187.

12. Ibid., 188.

13. Zachary Veilleux, "Better Sex, Naturally," *Men's Health,* November 1998, 140.

14. Ibid., 140.

15. Ibid., 140.

16. Ibid., 140.

17. Ibid., 142.

18. Ibid., 142.

19. Ibid., 142.

20. Ibid., 142.

Chapter Nine

Sexual Problems Women Encounter

1. Carlson Wade, *Nutritional Healers,* (West Wyack, NY: Parker Publishing Company, Inc., 1987), 191.

2. Ibid., 192.

3. Ibid., 192.

4. Michael T. Murray, N.D., *Healing Power of Herbs,* (Rocklin, CA: Prima Publishing, 1995), 375.

5. Ibid., 375.

6. Ibid., 375.

7. Ibid., 375.

8. Ibid., 376.

9. Ibid., 376.

10. Michael Murray, N.D. and Joseph Pizzorno, N.D., *Encyclopedia of Natural Medicine,* (Rocklin, CA: Prima Publishing, 1991), 525.

11. Ibid., 525.

12. Ibid., 528.

13. Ibid., 528.

14. Ibid., 530.

15. Ibid., 359.

16. Ibid., 530.

17. Ibid., 530.

18. Ibid., 532.

19. Ed Wheat, M.D. and Gaye Wheat, *Intended For Pleasure,* (Old Tappan, NJ: Fleming H. Revell Company, 1977), 110.

20. Ibid., 114.

Chapter Ten

Exercising to Enhance Your Sex Life

1. Dr. N. W. Walker, D.Sc., *Health, Happiness, and Longevity,* (Phoenix, AZ: O'Sullivan Woodside & Company, 1984), 140.

2. Ibid., 140.

3. Carlson Wade, *Nutritional Healers,* (West Nyack, NY: Parker Publishing Company, Inc., 1987) 152.

4. Michael Oppenheim, M.D., *The Men's Health Book,* (Englewood Cliffs, NJ: Prentice-Hall, Inc., 1994), 54.

5. *Mosby's Medical Dictionary,* s.v."Pubococcygeus exercises," (St. Louis, MO: Mosby Year Book, Inc., 4th ed., 1994).

Chapter Twelve

They Shall Be One Flesh

1. *Sex: A User's Manual,* (New York, NY: Berkley Publishing Corp., 1981) 103.

2. Ibid., 103.

3. Ed Wheat, M.D. & Gaye Wheat, *Intended For Pleasure,* (Old Tappan, NJ: Fleming H. Revell Company, 1977), 81.

4. *Sex: A User's Manual,* 106.

5. Ibid., 130.

6. Ibid., 134.

7. Ibid., 138.

8. Ibid., 140.

9. Ed Wheat, M.D.& Gaye Wheat, *Intended For Pleasure,* 87.

10. Ibid., 87.

11. Ibid., 87.

Chapter Thirteen

Foods, Thoughts and Sexual Performance

1. David C. Gardner, Dr. & Grace Joely Beatty, Dr., *Never Be Tired Again!* (New York, NY: Harper Perennial, 1990), 33.

2. Ibid., 33.

3. Ibid., 34.

4. Ibid., 37.

5. Ibid., 38.

6. Ibid., 39.

7. Ibid., 31.

8. Ibid., 31.

9. Ibid., 26.

10. Carlson Wade, *Magic Minerals,* (West Nyack, NY: Parker Publishing Company, Inc., 1967) 26.

Epilogue

Shaping Your Love Life

1. Michael L. McCann, Dr., *Secrets Of Self-Confidence In Christ,* (Middlesex, England: Zoe Publishing Company Ltd., 1989), IV.

2. Ibid., IV.

Printed in the United States
17717LVS00006B/283-360